Plantifully
Lean

D1210862

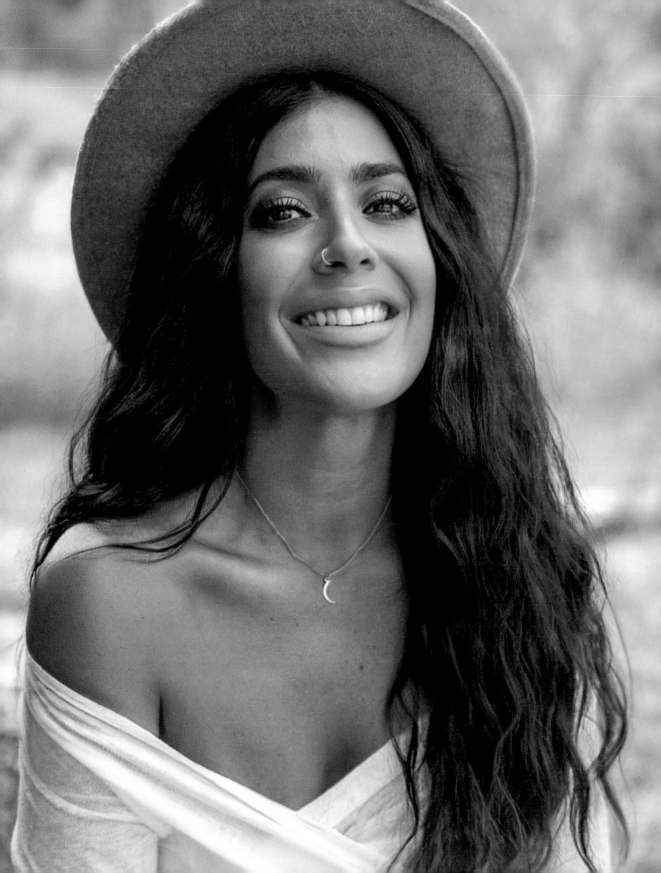

Plantifully
Lean

125+ Simple and Satisfying Plant-Based
Recipes for Health and Weight Loss

KIKI NELSON

SIMON ELEMENT

NEW YORK LONDON TORONTO SYDNEY NEW DELHI

SIMON
ELEMENT

An Imprint of Simon & Schuster, Inc.
1230 Avenue of the Americas
New York, NY 10020

Copyright © 2020 by Plantiful Living, LLC
Revised edition copyright © 2021 by Mountain Chi, LLC
Revised edition copyright © 2023 by Caroline Nelson
Originally published in 2020 by Plantiful Living, LLC

This publication contains the opinions and ideas of its author. It is intended to provide
helpful and informative material on the subjects addressed in the publication. It is sold with the
understanding that the author and publisher are not engaged in rendering medical, health, or any
other kind of personal professional services in the book. The reader should consult his or her medical,
health, or other competent professional before adopting any of the suggestions in this book or
drawing inferences from it.

The author and publisher specifically disclaim all responsibility for any liability, loss, or risk, personal
or otherwise, that is incurred as a consequence, directly or indirectly, of the use and application of
any of the contents of this book.

All rights reserved, including the right to reproduce this book or portions thereof in any form
whatsoever. For information, address Simon Element Subsidiary Rights Department,
1230 Avenue of the Americas, New York, NY 10020.

This Simon Element trade paperback edition April 2023

SIMON ELEMENT is a trademark of Simon & Schuster, Inc.

For information about special discounts for bulk purchases, please contact
Simon & Schuster Special Sales at 1-866-506-1949 or business@simonandschuster.com.

The Simon & Schuster Speakers Bureau can bring authors to your live event. For more information or
to book an event, contact the Simon & Schuster Speakers Bureau at
1-866-248-3049 or visit our website at www.simonspeakers.com.

Interior design by Allison Chi

Manufactured in the United States of America

1 3 5 7 9 10 8 6 4 2

Library of Congress Cataloging-in-Publication Data has been applied for.

ISBN 978-1-6680-1708-1
ISBN 978-1-6680-1709-8 (ebook)

For all the beautiful souls who have struggled with their weight and health, you are valuable and capable. Let's do this!

Contents

Welcome to Plantifully Lean

Hi and welcome! I adopted a high-carbohydrate, low-fat, plant-based diet after many failed attempts to lose weight and recover my health, and it was just the medicine I needed. I lost seventy pounds in a little more than a year. My life has never been the same.

I'm a wife and mother raising two beautiful kids in the Colorado mountains. I share my family life and health journey with plant-based eating and weight loss on YouTube and Instagram, where I'm known as "Plantiful Kiki." There, and as the co-creator of the Eat More Weigh Less Program, I aim to inspire others to regain their health, lose weight, and change their lives with simple and wholesome plant-based eating. I have found balance and joy in this lifestyle and I hope to impart some of that to you. I know how it feels to be overweight, and powerless to change it. At my heaviest, I carried 194 pounds on my petite five-foot-three frame. I had high blood pressure, high cholesterol, and high triglycerides, and I was prediabetic. I was at risk for stroke and a heart attack. No matter how hard I tried, I was never able to lose any significant amount of weight and turn around my health.

In other words, I was like most people—not at all good at losing weight. I would start a diet and an extreme exercise program only to "fall off the wagon" a few weeks in. When I did stick with a program for a few months, I would lose only a few pounds. The hard work and deprivation never seemed quite worth it. I was perpetually frustrated and constantly discouraged.

Everything changed when I found my way to a whole food plant-based diet. Once I learned the mechanics of weight loss and the fundamentals of calorie density, something finally clicked. The weight began to fall off.

It did not require calorie counting.

I did not have to eat less.

I did not go on an extreme exercise regimen.

I was free from the terrible cycle of depriving and binging and from calorie counting.

I learned how to build meals with delicious, filling foods, and I finally lost weight. At last, it wasn't so hard. What I learned and what I hope to teach you is that you can *eat more and weigh less*. In these next chapters, I will equip you with the basic tools and knowledge, along with the practical tips you will need to successfully lose weight and keep it off with little effort or thought. The information in this book is meant to be easy to understand and simple to apply.

It just takes some self-love—and a little bit of preparation to change your diet along with your outlook.

Let's do this!

Keep food
and life simple . . .
it multiplies
happiness.

Everything
you need *already*
lives *within* you.

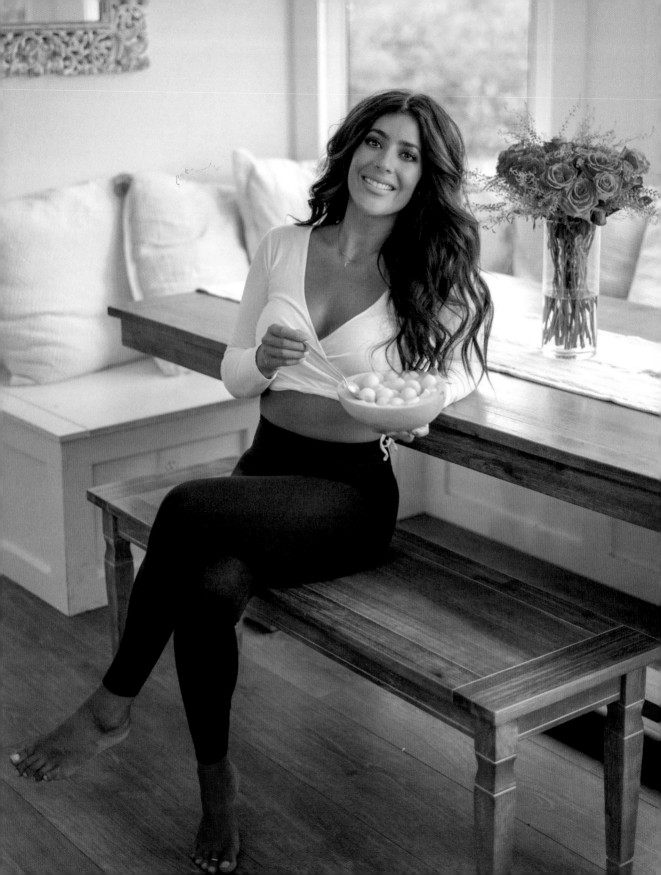

PART

1

The Mechanics of Weight Loss

How Weight Loss Works

Weight loss is simple, but it never *seems* easy.

In the following chapters you will learn that it *can actually be easy.*

You've likely heard that weight loss has to do with "calories in versus calories out." This is referred to as energy balance: the number of calories you take in versus the number of calories you use. So if I take in 3,000 calories a day but use only 2,200, then the excess 800 calories will be stored on my body as fat and I will gain weight.

While this is true, it's not *all the way* true. Our bodies metabolize calories from fat differently than they do calories from carbohydrates.

Carbohydrates are our body's preferred fuel source. If we consume an excess of calories from carbohydrates, our bodies store it in our muscles as glycogen, and the rest is burned off as body heat. This process is called thermogenesis. If we continue to consume a significant excess of calories from carbohydrates than what our body can use or burn off, it then starts the process of converting the carbohydrates to fat in a process called de novo lipogenesis (DNL).

Our bodies are not efficient at converting carbs to fat, and in fact we actually *burn calories* in order to convert carbohydrates. Fat, however, does not get converted to energy, or anything else for that matter. So, the excess calories from *fat* go straight to your "problem area." Reducing fat intake, rather than carbs, is one of the *major* reasons I was so successful in not only losing weight but also keeping it off.

The next time you hear someone tell you to avoid carbohydrates in food because "carbs turn to fat," recognize that this statement is a gross overexaggeration of the truth, is biologically inaccurate, and demonstrates a fundamental lack of understanding of human biochemistry and human biogenetics.
—Cyrus Khambatta, PHD, and Robby Barbaro, MPH,
Mastering Diabetes

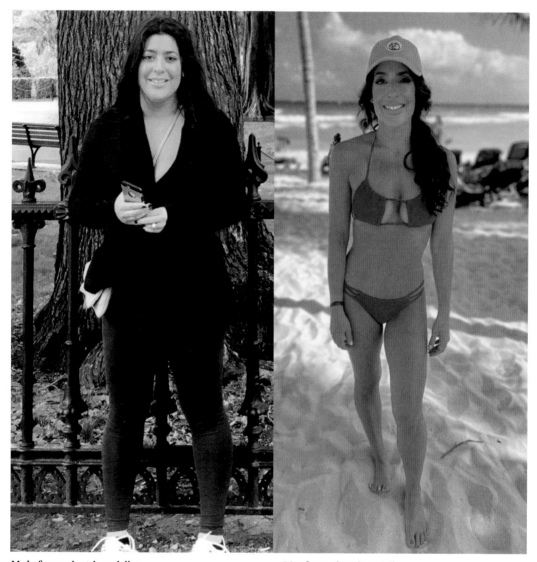

Me before a plant-based diet.   Me after a plant-based diet.

Calorie Density

Understanding calorie density is the most important tool you will have to guide you when making decisions regarding what to eat. Calorie density is simply the measure of energy, or calories, in a given amount of food. In this book, I will be talking about calories per pound. If you are anywhere else in the world, you will use calorie density in calories per kilogram. The same principles apply.

For example:
Broccoli has around 150 calories per pound.
Chocolate has around 3,000 calories per pound.

You want to eat foods that have fewer calories per pound. You can eat more of that food and feel full with fewer calories. Just think: A plate of broccoli and whole-grain pasta will fill you up, and you won't be accumulating excess calories. A big slice of cake may also fill you up, but you will be taking in a huge amount of calories.

Calorie density does not mean that you are counting calories. There is nothing I enjoy less. But I recognize that counting calories makes some people feel confident in how they choose foods, and if that's you, then by all means keep doing it. That's why I provide the calorie and macronutrient breakdowns in each recipe.

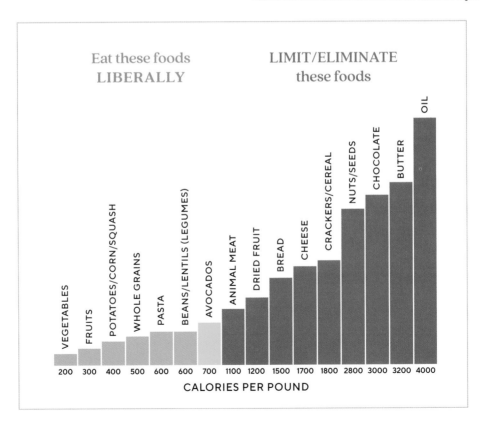

Eat these foods
LIBERALLY

LIMIT/ELIMINATE
these foods

VEGETABLES 200 · FRUITS 300 · POTATOES/CORN/SQUASH 400 · WHOLE GRAINS 500 · PASTA 600 · BEANS/LENTILS (LEGUMES) 600 · AVOCADOS 700 · ANIMAL MEAT 1100 · DRIED FRUIT 1200 · BREAD 1500 · CHEESE 1700 · CRACKERS/CEREAL 1800 · NUTS/SEEDS 2800 · CHOCOLATE 3000 · BUTTER 3200 · OIL 4000

CALORIES PER POUND

As Jeff Novick, MS, RDN, says in his video "Calorie Density: How to Eat More, Weigh Less, and Live Longer," people who eat mostly foods that are below the 600-calories-per-pound mark lose weight and are able to get into a healthy weight range. In the chart at left, I've highlighted all the foods that are 600 calories per pound or less in green, avocados in yellow, and other calorie-dense foods in red so that you make sure to eliminate them or eat them very sparingly as you journey toward your weight-loss goals.

But Who Cares?

I know what you're thinking: Who cares how many calories are in a pound of broccoli or in a pound of chocolate? I'm not eating a whole pound of chocolate in one sitting, so why does the calorie density matter?

It matters because people generally eat the same amount, or weight, of food each day, *regardless of the types of food* they eat.[1] So, again, if you want to lose weight successfully, the way to do it is not to eat less food but rather to eat the *same amount of food*—but make it food that has fewer calories.

Obese people have more energy-dense dietary patterns than healthy-weight individuals. In one survey, very obese men and women in the United States not only ate lots of energy-dense foods (big portions of meats, full-fat milk and cheese, fried eggs, high-fat desserts) but also very few low-energy-dense foods (salads, fruit, skim milk). Dutch researchers found that lean people have diets of lower energy density than obese people. The message is clear: "Eating a high-energy-dense diet is associated with elevated body weight."[2]

What matters for you is what happens when you *lower the caloric (energy) density of your daily meals.* According to this research, it doesn't really matter if you eat donuts all day or beans and rice all day. You need the same amount of food to feel satisfied. When it comes to feeling satiated, you will eat the same weight of food, regardless of the types of food you eat. So if you lower the caloric density of your meals, you will instantly start consuming fewer calories, resulting in effortless weight loss. But you won't feel hungry.

It's important to remember that the amount of food we need daily is unique to our individual biology. Your body craves its own specific amount of food, and your hunger drive will compel you to get that amount each day, which is why lowering the caloric density of your meals results in weight loss. I have seen it over and over in the thousands of individuals I have helped, as well as in my own life: Learning to eat according to calorie density is the magic pill you've been looking for, although it is no pill. It takes understanding these simple principles and then applying them.

You can do it. You are worth it.

And did I say: You won't feel hungry.

---

1   Barbara Rolls, PhD, and Robert A. Barnett, *The Volumetrics Weight-Control Plan* (New York: Harper, 1999), 17, 18.
2   Ibid.

Satiation

Let's face it: Not all foods are created equal. Some will satisfy us, while others leave us hungry soon after eating them.

Satiation is driven by several factors: calories, nutrients, and food weight. The combination of all these components influences whether you feel full. If your meal has calories and nutrients but not enough bulk or weight, you won't feel satisfied. This is why eating a small meal replacement bar might check all the calorie and nutrient boxes but leave you feeling hungry—it doesn't have the bulk/weight to trigger that nice feeling of not being hungry.

Here's a visual example of calorie density and satiation:

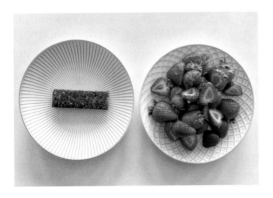

The plate on the left holds fruit leather, and the plate on the right holds fresh strawberries. Both have 120 calories. The fruit leather is just fruit that has been pureed and dehydrated, but the process has removed the fiber and water that add bulk and fill you up. The calories are still there; they've just been condensed. Now, I don't know about you, but that is not going to fill me up. But for the same calories, I can eat a whole bowl full of fresh strawberries that will satisfy me.

Why It Matters

If my hunger is driving me to eat four pounds of food, and I choose to eat foods that are high in calorie density each day, I'm likely to take in more calories than I need to eat to feel full, making weight loss impossible and weight gain probable.

Here's another way to think about it: *If the four pounds of food I eat one day consists of a food that contains 900 calories per pound, then another with 1,400 calories per pound, another with 1,800 calories per pound, and another with 850 calories per pound, then I've just consumed 4,950 calories in one day.* My body needs only about 2,000 calories daily to maintain its weight. This is why I was overweight for so many years. It wasn't my hormones or my genetics, or even my lack of exercise. It was the calorie density of the foods I was eating. The number of calories per pound matters.

How Does Weight Loss Actually Work?

To lose weight, you have to create a calorie deficit—there's just no way around it. I've tried every diet, even fad diet pills, that promised weight loss, but after years of broken promises, it still came down to the good old calorie deficit. After all that, I told myself I would never count calories again! And that's why calorie density is such a beautiful thing—it will carry you through your weight-loss journey without your ever having to track a single calorie. Eating according to the calorie-density principle makes you aware of whether you're consuming high-calorie foods without the need for painstaking calorie counting.

You Don't Have to Change Your Entire Diet!

Don't be overwhelmed by the thought of overhauling your diet. If you need to work your way into change, start by making over just one meal at a time. There's no shame in taking it slowly. Once you've conquered breakfast and have that routine down . . . then start making over lunch, and so on. This way, you can adjust as you build new habits that will last you a lifetime.

Calorie Dilution

When people consistently eat foods that are below 600 calories per pound, they lose weight—but there is a range to a healthy weight. Some individuals land at the top of a healthy weight range, some in the middle, and some at the lower end. Most of us want to fall at whatever point in that healthy weight range we perceive ourselves to look our best. For those who think their best is at the lower end of that range, the principles of calorie density make it possible to continue to eat the same volume of food one is used to while continuing to experience weight loss.

Cut the Calories, Not the Volume

This is where the real magic happens! I get so excited every time I have the opportunity to teach this, because it is so simple and can be so life-changing—it was for me! It is weight loss without deprivation.

Okay, let's say you have a big, beautiful bowl of pasta that has 700 calories. You then add ½ cup of marinara for 100 calories. The grand total for your meal is 800 calories. But let's say you're trying to lose those last unwanted pounds. Traditional diets mean restriction, small portions, and lots of hunger and moodiness to follow. (Just ask my husband how moody I got when I went low-carb!) But with calorie density, you get to *eat the same volume of food you did before you were dieting, but with fewer calories!* And here's how you do it.

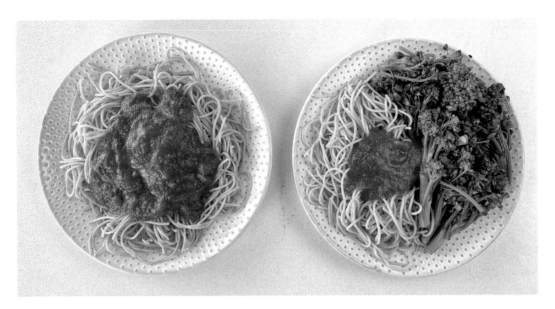

These two plates hold the same volume of food, but the one on the left has 800 calories and the one on the right has 500.

To dilute the calories of this dish without reducing the volume of food, you simply remove half the pasta and sauce and replace it with a steamed nonstarchy vegetable. Voilà—same volume, fewer calories!

For example, swap in some broccoli, and you now have 350 calories of pasta, 50 calories of marinara, and 100 calories of broccoli, for a grand total of 500 calories.

You were able to cut the calories of your meal nearly in half without reducing the amount of food. Plus, you get the added bonus of all the nutrition and bulk of the broccoli to help keep you full longer. This is what I affectionately call the $\frac{50}{50}$ plate. But there are other plate formulations. Read on!

How to Build Your Plate

There are **three** basic rules when it comes to building your weight-loss plate for every meal:

1. **Eliminate (or at least greatly reduce) added fats** from avocado, nuts, seeds, and nut and seed butters. Avoid all oils except where a light spray is necessary.

2. **Focus on whole, plant-based foods.** Avoid processed and calorie-dense packaged foods like crackers, chips, cookies, etc.

3. **Choose the plate that's best for you and build each meal accordingly.** If you want seconds, then serve yourself the same way, and always start with your veggies. This way, you are filling up on the least calorie-dense foods.

Plate 1: The ³⁰⁄₀ Plate

The ³⁰⁄₀ plate is great for someone who is just starting a plant-based, low-fat diet or who has a significant amount of weight (thirty pounds or more) to lose.

You will fill one-third of any size plate (hopefully a large one—I use a ten-inch dinner plate) with any nonstarchy vegetables, like steamed broccoli or roasted asparagus, then fill the remaining two-thirds of the plate with starches of your choice, such as baked potatoes, steamed rice, or whole-grain pasta. Remember to always eat your veggies first. Once your weight loss has slowed or stopped while using plate 1, you're ready to move down to the ⁵⁰⁄₀ plate. As you lose weight, your body needs fewer calories, and you can comfortably eat more nonstarchy vegetables and fewer starches.

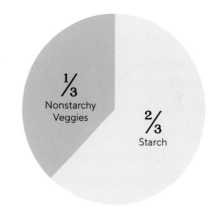

$\frac{1}{3}$ Nonstarchy Veggies

$\frac{2}{3}$ Starch

Plate 2: The $^{50}\!/_{50}$ Plate

The $^{50}\!/_{50}$ plate is the one I used to move past my weight-loss plateau all the way down to my current weight. This is also how I maintain my weight, and it's the plate most people will use to lose all the weight they are hoping to lose—and keep it off. For this plate, simply fill half your plate with nonstarchy vegetables and the other half with starches. And remember: Always eat your nonstarchy veggies first!

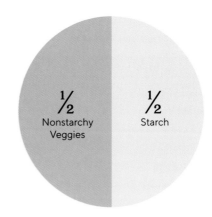

Plate 3: The $^{70}\!/_{30}$ Plate

The $^{70}\!/_{30}$ plate is not recommended for beginners or for weight maintenance. Rather, it's most useful when it comes to those last five to ten pounds. I like to refer to these as "vanity weight"—those pounds aren't detrimental to your health, but you might want to shed them to feel a little better or more comfortable with how you look. If the $^{50}\!/_{50}$ plate doesn't get you there, then this is the plate to move to. Once you've achieved your weight-loss goals, then you may move back up to the $^{50}\!/_{50}$ plate for weight maintenance (more on this later). (And as always, remember to eat your veggies first.)

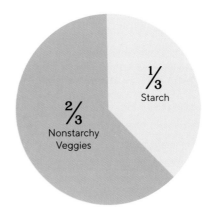

Adjusting to the ⁵⁄₅₀ Plate

AT FIRST, YOU MAY FEEL FULL *AND* HUNGRY

When I first started using the ⁵⁄₅₀ plate, I felt so full, but so hungry! Weird, right?

Here's what is happening: You are now taking in at least the same volume of food but way fewer calories than you used to. When you're losing weight, it is normal to feel some hunger, because you have to create a calorie deficit, and that's what this plate-building method helps you do.

You should not feel famished, however. If you feel really hungry, then by all means, eat! And I mean it! Have some fresh fruit or cut-up vegetables to tide you over until mealtime, and if that doesn't help, go ahead and eat something more substantial like a steamed potato with some cheese sauce (see page 176). Eat foods with fiber, water, and bulk, but not calories.

It can take your body a week or two to adjust, but hang in there, eat when you're hungry, and enjoy the journey.

YES TO PASTAS AND (SOME) BREAD!

Whole-grain pasta has a lower calorie density than other refined grain products like breads, crackers, and cookies, sitting at around 600 to 650 calories per pound, about the same as legumes. Whole-grain pasta digests slowly, which makes it a great option for the base of a healthy meal, especially when combined with plate-building principles.

Bread has a higher calorie density, with around 1,500 calories per pound, and gets digested quickly, so I recommend using sprouted whole-grain bread. It's full of fiber and will not digest as quickly as white bread. But sprouted or not, bread is still calorie dense, so be careful not to use it as the main source of calories for the majority of your meals.

MOSTLY AVOID: AVOCADOS, NUTS, AND SEEDS

Avocados, nuts, and seeds are extremely delicious and are healthy whole foods. But they're very calorie dense, with around 3,000 calories per pound, so to maximize weight loss, they should be eaten sparingly.

I use nuts and seeds more like toppings instead of eating them by the handful as a snack. Try sprinkling some on your oatmeal, salads, or nice creams, or just enjoy them in the dressings and sauces in this book that include them. Steer clear of full-fat nut butters and opt instead for low-fat powdered nut butters like PB2.

When it comes to avocado, you can be a little more liberal, because at right around 700 calories per pound, its calorie density is lower.

AVOID: PROCESSED FOODS, ANIMAL PRODUCTS, AND OILS

Processed Foods

Chips, crackers, and cookies are calorie-dense and low in nutrition. At best, they'll slow down weight loss, but it's most likely they'll simply prevent it. The only packaged foods I eat are sprouted bread, pasta, tortillas, and certain condiments, because they are part of recipes that are low in calorie density. They're also good for lunches. Of course, you can completely omit these items, if you wish, and focus on whole foods instead. Just remember that you want this journey to be enjoyable so it will be sustainable for you in the long term. If that means eating tortillas with some meals and adding wing sauce to others, I'm all for it. The most important thing is to stay on track and eat better than you used to—I'm for progress, not perfection!

Chocolate

I would never ask anyone to give up chocolate. Chocolate is a slippery slope, though. It's calorie-dense, with around 3,000 calories per pound, and it's also very high in fat. I sprinkle chocolate on fruit or use unsweetened cocoa powder to make chocolate desserts because you get more chocolate flavor for fewer calories and less fat.

Animal Products

Animal products like meat, cheese, milk, yogurt, and butter are all very high in fat, calories, and cholesterol, and should be minimized if not eliminated entirely for the best weight-loss results. If you're just starting your plant-based journey and still including some animal products, that's okay! Don't beat yourself up . . . just keep working toward increasing the amount of whole, fresh, plant-based foods you're eating.

Oils

Oils should be drastically reduced, if not completely eliminated from your diet. If you're new to this concept and find the taste of food unpalatable without it, try using a light spray of avocado oil. A little goes a long way for flavor, and enjoying your food goes an even longer way toward sustaining your new way of eating. A light spray here and there on your veggies or potatoes (or even on your popcorn to help seasonings stick) will not ruin your weight loss.[3] The things that slow or stop weight loss are

weekend junk food binges and overconsumption of more calorie-dense foods like chocolate, cookies, breads, crackers, and other processed foods. These can of course be enjoyed, but in moderation, so they don't stop your weight loss.

Starter Shopping List: Foods with 600 Calories or Fewer per Pound

(This list is not exhaustive, but it should give you a great place to start.)

GREENS

All greens are fantastic nutrient-dense foods. These are some of my favorites, but enjoy any greens you love, even if they aren't mentioned here.

Arugula	Parsley
Basil	Romaine lettuce
Cilantro	Spinach
Collard greens	Swiss chard
Kale	

NONSTARCHY VEGETABLES

Nonstarchy vegetables provide volume to your meals in addition to fiber, vitamins, and minerals. There are so many delicious nonstarchy vegetables to choose from. If you like only a few, that's okay. Choose the ones you love, and, over time, start venturing out and trying new ones.

Artichoke	Brussels sprouts
Asparagus	Cabbage
Bell pepper	Cauliflower
Bok choy	Celery
Broccoli	Cucumber

---

3 Using ⅛ to ¼ teaspoon of toasted sesame oil in Asian dishes adds a lot of flavor for little to no impact on weight loss. I note this as optional in a few recipes. You can choose to include it or leave it out.

Green beans

Mushrooms

Onions

Spaghetti squash

Summer (yellow)
  squash

Tomato

Zucchini

Oats, rolled or steel-
  cut (stay away from
  refined instant
  oats—they do not
  keep you full)

Popcorn

Quinoa

Rice, brown or white

Rice pasta

Whole-grain pasta

STARCHY VEGETABLES

Starchy vegetables will be the source of most of your calories. They provide vital energy and lots of satiation. Choose your favorites and enjoy. (My favorites are potatoes and beans.)

Acorn squash

Beans

Beets

Butternut squash

Carrots (can be
  used as a non-
  starchy vegetable in
  moderation)

Corn

Green peas (can
  be used as a non-
  starchy vegetable in
  moderation)

Lentils

Sweet potatoes

White potatoes

FRUIT

Fruit adds volume to your breakfast and makes a satisfying dessert. It's full of water, fiber, and nutrients that will help hydrate and nourish your body. Enjoy a wide variety of nature's candy.

Apples

Bananas

Berries

Cantaloupe

Cherries

Grapes

Honeydew

Mangoes

Oranges

Papaya

Peaches

Pears

Pineapple

Watermelon

GRAINS

Whole grains are filling and satisfying and make a great starchy option for your meals. I love oats, rice, whole grain pasta, and popcorn the most!

Amaranth

Barley

Millet

The brands in the lists that follow are the ones I reach for to build my plate because they are low in calorie density and delicious. But everyone has their own preferences, so feel free to swap brands or ingredients—just be mindful of the differences in calorie density and adjust accordingly.

Low-Calorie Tortillas and Wraps: Olé Mexican Foods Xtreme Wellness tortillas and wraps (available at any grocery store or Walmart); Joseph's Bakery lavash bread/wraps (available at any grocery store, Walmart, or Trader Joe's).

Sprouted Whole-Grain Bread: Ezekiel 4:9 sprouted bread (any variety) is around 80 calories per slice. This is usually kept in the freezer section at most grocery stores or Whole Foods. If you cannot find this brand, opt for another sprouted whole-grain bread; just be mindful of the calories. And if all else fails, opt for regular whole-grain bread.

Oil-Free Crackers: Edward & Sons brown rice crackers. I find these in most regular and natural grocery stores. They're oil-free and extremely crunchy!

Vegan Bouillon: Edward & Sons Not-Chick'n bouillon cubes. These are available at most grocery stores and at Whole Foods. The cubes do have some oil; to make them oil-free, prepare the broth according to the package instructions and refrigerate it overnight. In the morning, the fat will have hardened at the top, so you can remove it easily and still get all the flavor for your soups!

Plant Milks: I use thicker, higher-calorie milks (about 100 calories per cup) in dressings to yield a creamier, less watery dressing. I especially like Westsoy plain, unsweetened soy milk and Three Trees Organics plain, unsweetened almond milk. You can, of course, use whatever milk you enjoy; just know it can change the calorie counts of the dressings, as well as their consistency. If you want to use a low-calorie milk (about 30 calories per cup) or can't find the ones I recommend, simply add an additional ¼ cup raw cashews to the dressing before blending; this changes the calories per tablespoon by only a small amount. Almond Breeze plain, unsweetened almond milk (30 calories per cup) is great for Breakfast Berry Cereal (page 64) and if you like to add almond milk to your smoothies (see page 80) for extra creaminess and minimal added calories.

Gluten-Free Flour: I like Bob's Red Mill Gluten Free 1-to-1 Baking Flour. Where indicated, you can also use oat flour in place of regular flour.

Egg Replacer: Bob's Red Mill powdered gluten-free vegan egg replacer is my go-to. When adding egg replacer to a recipe, I don't bother to mix the powder with water; instead, I just throw it in with the dry ingredients. It's one less step.

Don't reduce your worth based on your *perception* of beauty . . . you *are* beautiful.

Why Go Plant-Based?

Why go plant-based? The answer is relatively simple: Animal products are full of fat and cholesterol and do not add to our overall well-being the way whole plant-based foods grown in nature do.

The thought of giving up all your favorite animal foods like cheese, butter, and bacon can be daunting. But here are five research-backed reasons that convinced me to give up animal products—they may make you want to transition to a plant-based diet, too.

1. Longevity

I'm fascinated by the Blue Zones. The residents of these five small pockets around the world (Okinawa, Japan; Sardinia, Italy; Nikoya, Costa Rica; Ikaria, Greece; and Loma Linda, California) have an unusually high life expectancy—one hundred years or more—and some of the lowest rates of the diseases that afflict people elsewhere, especially in North America.

Dan Buettner, a National Geographic Fellow and the *New York Times* bestselling author of numerous books about longevity, identified the Blue Zones and found a commonality among the people who live in these far-flung parts of the world: They eat a predominantly whole-food, plant-based diet that is low in fat.

2. Effortless Healthy Weight

I never used to believe in effortless weight balance. I thought there were those people who were blessed with skinny genes, and others, like me, who were not. Attaining and maintaining a healthy weight was a constant struggle for me. I felt like it was a battle I was always fighting. Then I came upon the work of Drs. John A. McDougall and Neal Barnard. In *The Starch Solution*, McDougall writes that the healthiest and trimmest people eat a low-fat, starch-based diet. He states: "Most people have been ingrained with the false notion, 'Don't eat starches, because starch turns to sugar, which turns to fat, making you gain weight.' If this were true, there would be an epidemic of obesity among the 1.73 billion Asians living on rice-based diets. After moving west and replacing their starch-based diet with animal foods, people from Japan and the Philippines would become trimmer and healthier. But that's not so. In fact, the opposite happens."[4]

I was terrified that I would gain more weight when I added carbs to my low-fat plant-based diet, but Dr. McDougall—and his experience helping thousands of people regain their health—convinced me that it was okay. To my absolute delight, I started seeing immediate results in my own health and weight. In just a month, I was no longer prediabetic, after having been prediabetic for years. Not only that but my cholesterol levels and blood pressure normalized, and I had lost ten pounds! All while eating plate-loads of carbohydrates.

---

4   John McDougall and Mary McDougall, *The Starch Solution* (New York: Rodale Books, 2013), 20.

3. Balanced Hormones

Hormone imbalance and hormone-related illnesses are rampant among Americans, and I was no exception. Popular diet culture tells us that we need high amounts of "healthy fats" in our diets to have good hormonal health, so I was religious about using organic unrefined coconut oil and grass-fed butter in my cooking. I bought pasture-raised eggs straight from the farm and cooked only grass-fed beef. But my health worsened over time, and I gained weight. I was plagued by horribly painful menstrual cycles and mystery spotting. My doctor said I was at very high risk for developing polycystic ovary syndrome (PCOS). I also had all the symptoms of hypothyroidism, including acne and hair loss. But as I continued to embrace my high-carb, low-fat plant-based diet, all these eventually resolved.

Dr. Neal Barnard has helped thousands of people reverse their health issues through low-fat plant-based diets, and his book *Your Body in Balance* has been an important resource and encourager for me along my weight-loss journey. He writes: "Some of the most serious conditions we face—weight problems, diabetes, and cancer of the breast, ovary, uterus, or prostate—are related to foods that are causing hormone haywire. And for less serious conditions—the health of your skin and whether you keep a full head of hair—hormones play a key role, too. Foods turn the dials on virtually every biological function."[5]

I learned from Dr. Barnard that a diet high in fat can increase estrogen levels, and, conversely, that if I really gave 100 percent to a low-fat plant-based diet, I could potentially reverse my painful menstrual cycles, not to mention whatever role my hormones could be playing in weight gain. In *Your Body in Balance*, he states: "When women change their diets, the amount of estrogen in their blood changes, too. While high-fiber foods tend to reduce estrogen levels, fatty foods do the opposite. They increase estrogens . . . To avoid excess fats, the first step is to skip animal products. This helps you avoid the worst actors, the saturated fats in dairy products and meat."[6]

These sentences further confirmed that eliminating fat from animal products and reducing my overall fat intake had been the right thing to do.

Between Dr. McDougall's call for satisfying carbs and Dr. Barnard's warnings about animal products, I immediately overhauled my diet to be plant-based and low-fat, and the results were not only amazing but freeing. I had struggled with my weight for so many years, and felt as if my health was slipping further away from me. To reclaim my well-being through my diet, something I could control, was the single most empowering experience of my life.

If you are struggling with your health or at risk for developing chronic issues, know that there is a solution. The work of these incredible doctors was my starting place, and I would point you in their direction, too. Don't give up, and don't give in. You deserve to live a healthy and vibrant life, and it is within your reach.

---

5 Neal D. Barnard, MD, with Lindsay Nixon, *Your Body in Balance: The New Science of Food, Hormones, and Health* (New York: Grand Central, 2020), xi.
6 Barnard and Nixon, *Your Body in Balance*, 40–41.

4. Prevent Sickness and Disease

As books on health and diet stacked up around me, one major theme appeared repeatedly: Declining health and rising disease are rooted in our modern diet and habits. An abundance of fatty, overprocessed, and chemical-laden foods has made it more challenging to simply choose only wholesome foods. The foods that are easy to prepare and convenient are full of fat and calories. Our health has declined, and obesity is at epidemic levels.

Dr. McDougall writes: "There is one fundamental difference between the danger of animal foods and that of cigarettes and drinking. With tobacco and alcohol, the risks are nearly universally understood. We know the facts. Meat, poultry, fish, seafood, cheese, milk, and eggs, on the other hand, are widely considered an appropriate, even essential part of a healthy diet. Most people eat these risky foods believing that they are nutritious and life sustaining. . . . We don't consider the danger inherent in eating these foods because nobody has told us how harmful they really are."[7]

The more I read the work of these respected doctors, the more apparent it became to me that if I was going to improve my health, my eating habits had to change. Once I began to change my eating habits, my health immediately started improving and I lost weight. Within months, my cholesterol, triglycerides, and blood sugar levels were in healthy ranges. My doctor couldn't believe that after struggling for so many years with my weight and health, I had come so far in just a few short months.

5. Mitigate Diabetes

The struggle with diabetes is something very near to my heart.

Type 2 diabetes runs deep in my family's history, and I've lost beloved family members to this all too common disease. For years, I was prediabetic; my fasting blood sugar was double the norm. Again, it was Dr. Neal Barnard who helped me understand what was really causing my insulin resistance, and what was keeping it alive. Sugar from carbohydrates doesn't cause insulin resistance, as I had believed—fat does! This was a huge revelation. I learned that it's the accumulation of tiny amounts of fat inside the muscle cells that makes it hard for insulin to do its job, by blocking what is called insulin signaling. That is, the fat interferes with the process by which insulin opens the cell membrane to allow glucose to enter.[8] In other words, a low-fat, plant-based diet full of whole foods promotes insulin sensitivity, which is exactly what people who are prediabetic and diabetic lack.

Sugar is your body's preferred fuel source, whether you choose to get it from whole starches, whole grains, fruit, or a combination thereof. Remember, diabetes doesn't result from too much sugar but rather an excess of fat.

---

7   McDougall, *Starch Solution*, 35.
8   Neal D. Barnard, MD, *Dr. Neal Barnard's Program for Reversing Diabetes: The Scientifically Proven System for Reversing Diabetes Without Drugs* (New York: Rodale Books, 2018), 41.

Eat More, Weigh Less: The Basics of Calorie Density

1

Eat foods below the 600-calories-per-pound mark. This includes foods such as potatoes, squash, rice, oats, and all varieties of fruits and vegetables (see page 16).

2

Eliminate oils for the quickest and biggest reduction in calories.

3

Use nuts, seeds, nut and seed butters, and avocado sparingly. You can use avocado more than nuts and seeds because its calorie density is 750 calories per pound versus about 3,000 calories per pound for nuts and seeds.

4

Avoid processed foods and eat vegetables, fruits, whole grains, and legumes.

Common Concerns About a Plant-Based Diet

What About Protein?

Some of the most common questions I receive are about protein. "How do I get enough protein?" "Do I need to track my protein intake?" "Is there enough protein in a plant-based diet?"

These are all great questions, and they have a simple answer: You will absolutely get enough protein on a plant-based diet. You do not need to focus on it or track it. Here's the thing: As a society, we've become obsessed with protein. We're being sold high-protein animal products, protein shakes, and protein bars, but the protein pitch is nothing but marketing. Just remember that all the longest-lived people on the planet eat a primarily plant-based diet.

There is protein in every plant food; beans, peas, lentils, asparagus, and broccoli are all excellent sources of plant protein.[9] As long as you eat a variety of plants—whole grains, legumes, vegetables, and seeds and nuts (these in lower amounts for weight loss)—so that you don't feel hungry or lethargic, you'll be getting enough protein. What's more, animal protein can be harmful; it contains sulfur, which interferes with the body's ability to maintain calcium and can even contribute to kidney failure. Plant proteins, however, are not harmful.

Am I Getting Enough Healthy Fats?

The idea that we need to consume all this added fat from oils or animal foods is sadly, again, just more marketing. The low-carb weight-loss industry sells us the idea that our bodies need fat as their fuel source when that is biologically inaccurate. Our bodies and brains run on sugar from carbohydrates. There is, however, fat in all plant foods—even lettuce, grains, beans, and legumes have trace amounts—and we do not need the amount of fat in our diets that we have been led to believe.[10] These small amounts of essential fats are perfectly packaged the way nature intended, with the natural fiber, sugars, proteins, vitamins, and minerals also found in the plant. In other words, as Dr. Neal Barnard explains, "You will never eliminate vegetable oils completely. There are always traces of natural oils in grains, beans, vegetables, and fruits, which supply the tiny amount of fat—about 3 to 4 percent of your calories—that your body needs."

What About Fruit?

Whole, fresh fruits are wonderful foods, full of fiber, water, and nutrients. Not only are they low

---

9   Neal A. Barnard, MD, *Turn Off the Fat Genes: The Revolutionary Guide to Losing Weight* (New York: Harmony, 2001), 121–22.
10   Ibid.

in calorie density, they also hydrate your skin, detoxify your body, and provide antioxidants and other antiaging nutrients.

Fruit makes a satisfying snack or dessert when you want something sweet. I love having a bowl of sliced fresh peaches at the end of a meal. A big serving of fresh berries alongside your oatmeal is a healthy way to start the day.

Over the years, I've found that the more fresh fruit I eat, the less junk I crave, and the leaner I become. When I snack on fruit, I'm less tempted by processed foods like cookies and crackers. Even better is that when I eat more fruit, I find that my skin is more hydrated and glowing.

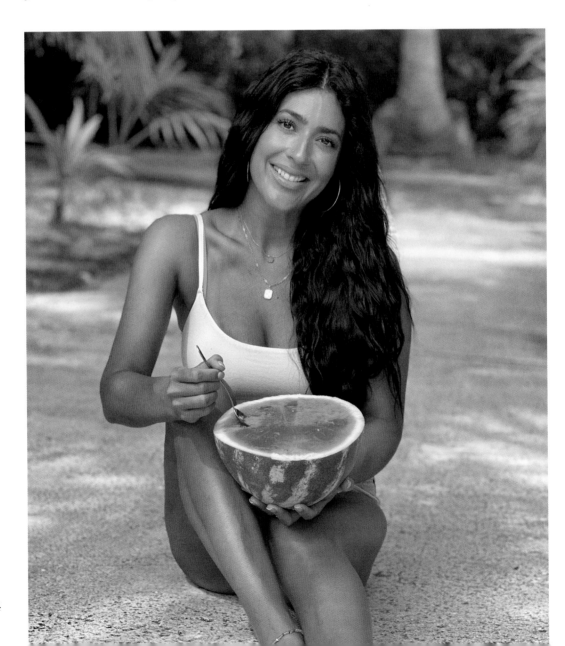

Troubleshooting Stubborn Weight

Sometimes those last few pounds just won't go away. If that stubborn weight is sticking to you, consider the following:

Keep diluting your calories. To further dilute calories, preload your meal and start with a vegetable soup or salad *before* moving on to your ⁵⁰/₀₀ plate.

In a study conducted by Dr. Henry Jordan, MD, at the University of Pennsylvania, participants were asked to eat soup at least four times a week. He found that the more soup participants ate, the more weight they lost, and that participants consumed an average of 100 fewer calories a day than those who ate soup less frequently.[11] This is the principle of calorie density at work. Fill up on the least calorie-dense foods first. They help keep you full and satisfied so you won't be tempted to eat a lot of calorie-dense foods.

If you're still hungry after your soup and ⁵⁰/₀₀ meal, go back for seconds, starting with more soup. Chances are, you'll be too full after that to eat another helping of the more calorie-dense side of your meal. The fiber and bulk will help keep you full, and you'll end up eating fewer calories throughout the day. If you do this consistently, you will likely see weight loss.

Make sure you're eating whole foods that are low in calorie density. The foods that are lowest in calorie density and highest in nutrition are plants. A whole-food, plant-based diet that is low in fat is naturally the diet with the lowest calorie density. You can eat large volumes of these foods for fewer calories than an equal volume of animal foods or any processed food. Not to mention that a plant-based diet is environmentally sustainable, great for health, and affordable, if you stick to simple whole foods like fruits, vegetables, whole grains, and starches and steer clear of expensive processed plant-based foods like plant-based meats and cheeses.

Double-check that you are minimizing the amount of overt fat you consume. This is key to successful weight loss. If you're having trouble losing weight, make sure you're no longer cooking with oil, and that you are being *very* moderate with your use of nuts and seeds (including nut and seed butters). You can be a little more liberal with avocado because it is not as high in calorie density.

Double-check that you are cutting out processed and packaged foods. This is also essential, especially if you tend to rely on them as a source of calories. Instead of snacking on chips, crackers, cookies, and breads, opt for fresh fruits and vegetables. Some of the recipes in this book include store-bought tortillas and whole-grain breads, but these shouldn't have a negative effect or derail your goals if you're eating them in moderation. But if you'd like to steer clear of *all* processed/packaged food, then stick to the recipes that don't include them or substitute something else in their place. It's all about making this lifestyle work for you so that you can have long-term success.

---

11   Rolls and Barnett, *Volumetrics Weight Control Plan*, 101.

FAQs

How much should I eat?

You can eat as much as you need to in order to feel satisfied. Don't let yourself feel hungry! Go back for seconds and thirds. Just keep serving yourself the same way (with a ⁵⁄₀₀ plate or one of the others on pages 13–14), and always eat your nonstarchy vegetables first. This will keep you filling up on the least calorie-dense foods and help prevent you from overeating the more calorie-dense starches. You'll find that after a second helping of vegetables, you're probably too full for another helping of starch.

What size plate should I use?

Any size is fine. I use a big 10-inch dinner plate or a large 9- to 10-inch serving bowl, but everyone is different. Some can eat more than others, and some less. I can eat more volume than my husband. Remember, it's not about restricting volume, it's about eating fewer calorie-dense foods, keeping it low-fat, and using one of the calorie dilution plate models like the ⁵⁄₀₀ plate (see page 14).

What about fruit at breakfast instead of vegetables?

I know it can feel unnatural to eat vegetables for breakfast, but I promise it gets easier. One day, you'll realize you can't imagine breakfast without them! Having a big serving of nonstarchy vegetables with breakfast will help keep you full and satisfied all morning. You can also try adding nonstarchy vegetables like mushrooms, onions, and bell peppers to omelets, breakfast burritos, and potato hash.

For those of you who can't stomach vegetables in the morning and prefer a sweet breakfast, have some fresh fruit before you enjoy your starch. Fruit is still very low in calorie density and very high in fiber, nutrients, and bulk, and will help fill you up. So enjoy a big bowl of berries or any other fruit you like.

Can I snack?

When it comes to snacking, just remember to keep it simple. Calories add up quickly, especially with foods like crackers, chips, and breads that are easy to overeat in a short amount of time. For the best weight loss results, stick to fresh veggies and any of the snacks in chapter 4. You can also snack on whole, fresh fruits. Snacking on processed foods will slow down your weight loss or, worse, stop it.

What about dessert?

Fruit is the best dessert for weight loss—not only is it sweet but it's also filling, nutritious, and full of fiber. I know that we all just need something a little decadent sometimes, which is why I've included a dessert recipe section (see chapter 5). As a general rule, try to stick with fruit or my "nice cream" (see pages 234–39) for dessert for most of the week, and then use the other dessert recipes for a special, more decadent dessert on the weekend.

What about alcohol and coffee (aka liquid calories)?

Water is best. You want to be mindful of consuming liquid calories; not only do they add up quickly, they also don't do much to make you feel full or satisfied. If you don't like drinking water, try making fancy spa water by adding chopped berries and cucumber to gently flavor it.

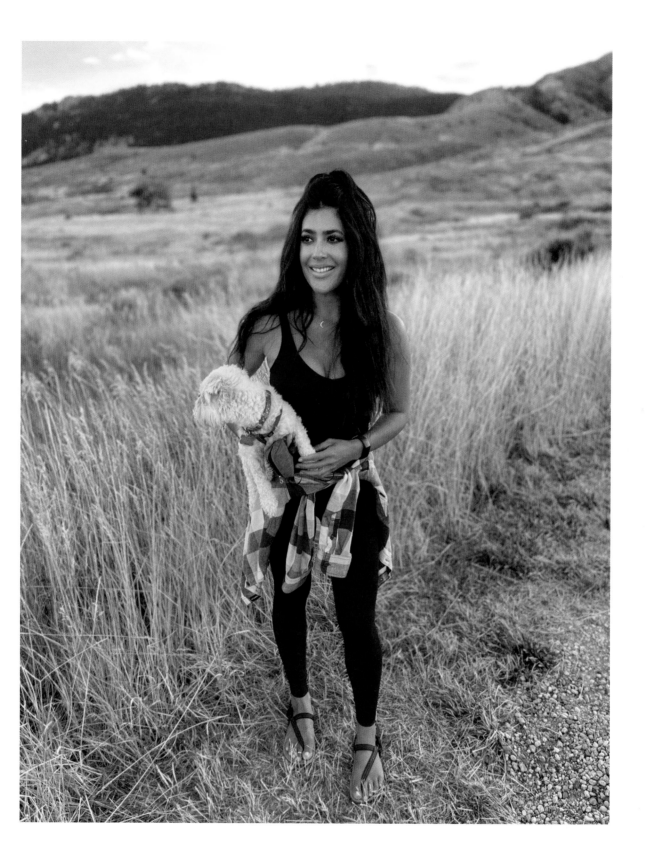

One cup of coffee a day is permissible, but don't fill it with fatty, high-calorie creamers and sweeteners. Instead, add almond milk and some French vanilla stevia to sweeten it.

Avoid alcohol. If you're out with friends, ask for a seltzer with a splash of your favorite fruit juice. When you're home and want something special to drink, try one of the sparkling stevia-sweetened drinks available like Zevia. I like to make a mock mojito by adding lime and crushed mint to a Zevia ginger ale!

What about sugar, syrups, and other sweeteners?
Refined sugars pack a lot of calories for little to no nutritional value, and do not help you feel full or satisfied. Instead, opt for all-natural sugar-free syrups and stevia or monk fruit for sweetening. Pure maple syrup in small amounts is also permissible, and it's okay to use small amounts of unrefined sugar.

What if I'm tracking calories?
Even though my claim to fame is helping individuals lose weight and keep it off without ever having to count calories, I know many people feel more comfortable tracking their calorie intake. For this reason, I've included nutrition information with calorie counts for each recipe. These counts are estimates generated by the nutrition calculator I use, based on the specific food items I select from the thousands of options in that calculator's database, the products I use, and my style of cooking and measuring ingredients. Use the nutrition info as a guideline, but remember that everyone cooks slightly differently.

If complete accuracy is important to you, I suggest using a nutrition calculator like Cronometer or MyFitnessPal to track what you eat by weight. For example, when you record the calories of potatoes, the most accurate reading will be based on the weight of the potatoes (such as 14 ounces/400 grams), not their volume (such as 2 cups). Absolute accuracy does not exist when it comes to tracking calories because there is variation in how we measure and what brand of ingredients we use, so it's more of an art than a science. It does, however, provide you with calorie ranges to reference, which can be very helpful.

But let me assure you once again that you can make great strides in losing weight by consistently applying the principles of calorie density along with the plate-building method—I've lost seventy pounds without ever counting a single calorie.

How to Maintain Your Weight Loss

Once you've reached your desired weight, maintaining it is simple. Stick with the ⁵⁄₁₀ plate for all your main meals, and eat the vegetables first. Keep snacking on veggies and fruit, and enjoy treats in moderate amounts.

Because maintaining your weight requires more calories than losing weight, you can enjoy more calorie-dense meals more frequently. When you've reached your weight loss goal, slowly reintroduce some healthy fats if you had previously cut them out. A good rule of thumb is no more than ¼ to ½ an avocado, ½ to 1 ounce of nuts and seeds, and 1 tablespoon of ground flaxseed a day. (Do not reintroduce oil to your cooking, except for the occasional spray here and there.) If your weight starts to go up, cut the amount of fat in half. Your body will tell you how much of these fats it will tolerate; listen to and work with your body. Keep an eye on the treat foods, stay consistent, and love yourself along the way.

Find Daily Movement You Enjoy

It's important to find some type of movement you enjoy and will look forward to enough to incorporate into your daily routine. I'm not a fan of extreme exercise programs (but if you are, go ahead and enjoy yourself!); this is all about finding movement that you enjoy. Walking outdoors is the most pleasurable form of daily exercise for me, and during my weight-loss phase, I took a brisk thirty-to-forty-minute walk every day. I still take a thirty-minute walk every single day because I love any opportunity to be outside in nature. I've also incorporated some weight lifting into my movement three days a week, but again, no extreme workouts for me.

Remember that exercise should be a reward, something that you look forward to and that brings you joy. It shouldn't be seen as a punishment for eating a super-calorie-dense meal or as a dreaded daily chore. Find the movement that makes you happy.

And if you have a sedentary job or you're physically unable to move, you can still make great progress without it.

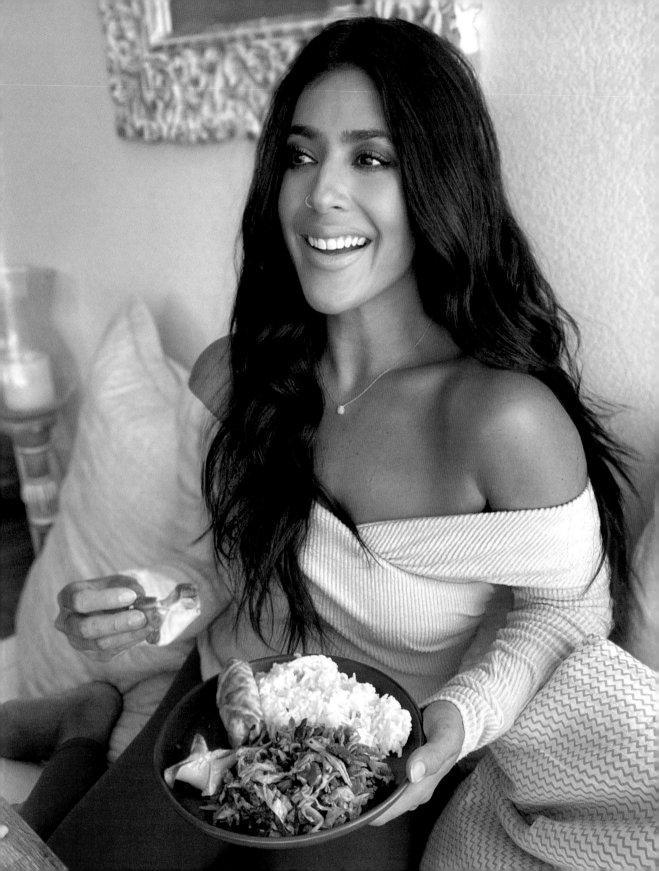

Getting Started

Self-Love Will Empower Lasting Change

Over the years, I've found that the answer to long-term success and change isn't discipline. It's more basic. Yes, discipline has its place, but it won't empower change in your life the way that self-love and compassion do. Self-love is the key to empowering change. When you embrace your worth and value, you begin to move through life the way you were intended to…full of joy and peace. Your choices become based on what is best for you, not what is easiest or what aligns with your negative feelings about yourself.

Believe You Deserve It

What you believe, you become. What you feel, you attract. What you imagine, you create.
—**Attributed to the Buddha**

That saying could not be more true. When I was younger, I struggled with self-worth, always comparing myself to others and believing I didn't have what it would take to change or be different. But over the years, as I embraced the truths of my innate self-worth, my life began to radically change.

The relationship you have with yourself directly impacts your ability to live a happy and fulfilling life, and your ability to dream and achieve. I hope with every fiber of my being that you find strength in this—that you find the encouragement and the empowerment to begin believing in your innate value and self-worth

as an individual—a worth that is not tied to a certain weight or age or arbitrary standard of beauty. All those things are subject to change. You, my love, have value that does not change. It is constant.

Your Value Is Constant

Your value does not change based on the opinions of others, or even on your own opinion of yourself. Your value is inherent. It's part of your humanity, and of the amazing and capable body your beautiful soul lives within. So start believing that you are remarkable, beautiful, and treasured—because you are.

Let It Sink In

No one can make you feel inferior without your consent.
—**Attributed to Eleanor Roosevelt**

Let that sink in. *No one* can take away your self-worth unless you let them. And that includes yourself!

When I started changing the way I talked to myself, my life started to change. I no longer accepted negative thoughts about myself. I would no longer participate in putting myself down, because I was growing to respect myself too much for that. And let me tell you something: In time, self-respect will grow into a deep self-love and appreciation. Make it a habit.

I Empathize

I understand what it's like to feel insecure, ugly, fat, and like I'm not enough. I understand the pain and anxiety that can accompany those thoughts and feelings, and I understand the loneliness they can bring. I'm here to tell you that you can heal your self-image and completely change your life as a result. If I can do it, you definitely can, too.

The Road to Self-Love

My journey of self-love was beautiful and non-linear, and I wouldn't change a thing. It took time and practice, but it completely changed my life. I'm sitting here writing this with so much joy because I have become a healed, happy, confident, joyful individual who believes she can do anything she puts her mind to. The road to self-love will wind forward and backward. It will feel beautiful and ugly. It will be freeing and frustrating. But if you understand the goal of learning to love yourself and why it's important, and you keep gently working at it, you will get there.

Here are the four areas that are harnessed along the path to self-love:

MINDSET

The mindset you carry about your body, your worth, your beauty, your importance, and your ability to be successful directly affects your ability to follow through and be consistent.

DISCIPLINE

Discipline is great and has its place, but it's actually fueled by your mindset and sense of self-worth.

I AM WHAT I BELIEVE

If I believe that I'm beautiful, that I'm valuable, that I'm worth taking care of, and that I can do anything I set my mind to, then I'm unstoppable!

Your issue really isn't how you look in clothes, how much you weigh, or even what others think about you. Your issue is what you believe about yourself.

PRACTICE CREATES CHANGE, NOT PERFECTION

The practice of self-love is what empowers change. When you practice loving yourself and believing in yourself, nothing can stop you! Does it mean you're perfect? Nope. It just means that you can't be defeated. Self-love is a practice. At first it feels like a muscle you haven't flexed much, if ever. It's going to feel awkward and unnatural. But, as with anything, practice and consistency will deliver results.

Practical Steps to Build Self-Love

You may be reading this not knowing where to start. Or you're thinking there's nothing you love about yourself, and that you can't even imagine practicing loving yourself. I've got you! I've been there, too. When I started my weight loss journey back to health, I was seventy pounds overweight, insecure, and anxiety-ridden. I couldn't come up with *anything* I loved about myself. So I started smaller: I made a list of the things I could *appreciate* about myself. Now, if you still can't think of a few things you can appreciate about yourself, then call your bestie and have them help you make this list. This list is your starting point, and you can't cross the finish line without it.

Step 1: List the things you can appreciate or love about yourself

Examples:

- I appreciate that my body made two healthy babies.
- I appreciate that my body has been there for me through every crash diet and crazy exercise routine I've put it through.
- I appreciate that I didn't die back in 2013 when I got the flu and thought I might actually die!
- I appreciate my thick hair.

Step 2: Make a list of affirmations— kind things to say to yourself that you may not believe now but certainly want to someday.

Examples:

- I am amazing.
- I am beautiful.
- I am smart.
- I am strong.
- Anything I can imagine, I can have.

Self-love will *always* move you
further than self-hate, because what
we love, *we take care of.*

READ THIS LIST EVERY MORNING AND EVERY NIGHT

What I'm about to tell you is the most important thing, after making your list. Every morning, as soon as you wake up, take five minutes and sit with yourself and your list in a quiet, private place. Do the same thing every evening, just before you go to bed. Look at your list and hold yourself (hug yourself), and repeat your affirmations and appreciations out loud to yourself. Even if you don't believe them right away, intend on one day believing them, and soon you'll find that your self-hate has turned into appreciation. Appreciation will grow into self-respect, and self-respect will grow into self-love.

You'll have good days and you'll have bad days. You'll have good moments and you'll have bad moments. But remember, you're looking for progress, not perfection. You'll start to realize that you don't talk to or about yourself the way you used to. You'll notice that you are more patient with yourself, more kind with yourself, and you will start to realize your true value and worth.

CELEBRATE THE SMALL WINS

This sounds silly, but it's super important: Every time you have a small win, applaud yourself with words of affirmation. Neuroscience confirms that these small celebrations and positive affirmations rewire your brain for success. When you celebrate small wins, you experience more self-confidence and joy. In the same way you praise your children or your dog to affirm their good habits and behavior, praise yourself. When you finish your affirmations in the morning, stand up and say, "Woohoo! I positively impacted my self-worth for the day," and give yourself a round of applause. I know it sounds silly, but this makes a huge difference in how fast you start to feel change.

Remember: Change takes time, and again, your aim is progress, not perfection. So relax. Don't worry if you don't believe what you're saying or if you're "feeling" different. It's the practice that moves you forward, not the flawless execution of it all. Healing takes time, and it can feel like you're taking two steps forward and one step back. Healing can be emotional, frustrating, and completely amazing all at the same time, so be patient with yourself. Speak kindly to yourself. You are giving yourself the biggest gift you could ever give: self-love.

You are beautiful.

How to Use the Recipes in This Book

Each recipe comes with the macronutrient and calorie breakdown so you can feel comfortable with what you eat. I've included the calorie counts, but you do not need to track calories to lose weight.

I've organized the recipe sections into Breakfast; Lunch and Dinner; Soups, Salads, and Sides; Snacks and Cravings; and Desserts.

The recipes in the Cravings section are there for the weekend when you feel like something special or you're really craving some takeout or fast food. These recipes require a little more effort and are a little more calorie-dense, but they're still fantastic for weight loss. And they're a great way to satisfy those cravings without giving in to convenience foods packed with processed ingredients, sugar, and tons of fat. It's important not to feel deprived—you still get to enjoy the weekend, so use these cleaned-up foods to satisfy you and keep you on track.

I generally eat simply and repetitively during the workweek, then plan for a more "fun weekend"-type meal to mix it up when I have a little more time. I always look forward to my cleaned-up vegetable pizza or Buffalo cauliflower wing salad along with a stack of blueberry vanilla pancakes for Saturday or Sunday breakfast. I believe these end-of-the-week Cravings dishes are what keep me from feeling deprived. I look forward to eating on the weekend without going all out on vegan junk food.

You decide which recipes appeal to you and make them accordingly.

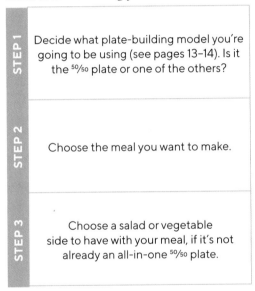

STEP 1	Decide what plate-building model you're going to be using (see pages 13–14). Is it the $^{50}/_{50}$ plate or one of the others?
STEP 2	Choose the meal you want to make.
STEP 3	Choose a salad or vegetable side to have with your meal, if it's not already an all-in-one $^{50}/_{50}$ plate.

The recipes that are a complete $^{50}/_{50}$ meal will be indicated by this icon: ⬤. If a recipe doesn't have this icon, then add a side of veggies to your plate to complete the $^{50}/_{50}$ meal.

For recipes that include fats from nuts, seeds, or avocados, these ingredients can, of course, be omitted and adjusted to be 100 percent fat-free. The choice is yours.

Tips for Success

Be Prepared

The old saying "If you fail to prepare, then you prepare to fail" rings true. Spend a little time every week shopping for groceries and getting some of your foods made ahead of time so your meals will be easier to prepare during the week (see "Prep Day," page 39). Stock up on items you'll need to make weekly meal prep easier.

Be Kind to Yourself

Self-compassion will always move you further than self-hate. Be kind and patient with yourself, especially when you mess up—because you will. It is not about perfection; it's just about consistently heading in the right direction.

Be Consistent

Consistency is also key to your success. When we're consistent all week but lose our composure on the weekends and go on those high-fat/high-calorie escapades, it can really stall or stop our progress. This is why I suggest choosing simple and repetitive meals during the workweek, and then going for meals from the recipe section like pizza or Buffalo cauliflower wings, and pancakes for the weekend. It helps you feel satisfied, allowing you to enjoy "weekend" foods while avoiding the junk food pitfalls.

Stay Low-Fat or Fat-Free

Avoid cooking with oil except for a light spray of avocado oil here and there to help keep things from sticking to a pan, or to help you as you transition to cooking without oil. There are a few recipes that call for $\frac{1}{8}$ to $\frac{1}{4}$ teaspoon of toasted sesame oil, because sesame oil adds a lot of flavor for a tiny amount of fat. You can omit it if you want to.

Eliminate nut and seed butters and instead enjoy the salad dressings and cheese sauce in this book, the latter of which contains just a small amount of nuts. Avocados are still very low in calorie density at around 750 calories per pound, so they can be enjoyed a little more liberally. If you find that you're not losing weight, consider eliminating overt fats altogether for a few weeks to see how your body responds. We all have a tendency to take in more calories than we realize.

Know Your Reason

Changing any major aspect of your life requires some discipline, and eating a plant-based, low-fat diet is no exception. Knowing *why* you're changing your routines and habits will help you make good decisions when you're tempted to eat foods with lots of fat or sugar, or when you're tired and want to reach for something convenient and likely processed. Don't be afraid to tell others, and yourself, that you're eating this way to meet your goals. You don't need to explain the science or your reasons, but politely ask that they respect what you are doing for yourself.

Move

Exercise is not necessary for weight loss when you're eating this way, but for your mental and physical well-being, it's always a good idea to move your body every day. During my weight-loss journey, I simply walked for thirty to forty minutes a day. That's all the exercise I did, and I still lost almost seventy pounds. If you love to exercise, then keep going; if you hate it, then try to find something you like to do, like taking a walk for at least twenty minutes a day. If you are too heavy or have joint issues and can't manage a walk, that's okay—you can still lose weight as long as you consistently stick to the rules of plate building.

When you start to lose weight, exercising will become more comfortable.

Get Support

Feeling supported will help you stay motivated and consistent. If your spouse or significant other doesn't want to jump on board, then find a friend. If you can't find a friend, then hop on social media and follow my accounts to see the motivational content I'm always sharing. You'll also find many other people there on the same journey. It's all about finding ways to stay motivated.

○ Plantifulkiki
○ Plantifulkiki
○ Plantifulkiki
○ Plantifulkiki

Rest

Make sure you rest. Get lots of sleep and spend a little time every day doing something you love, whether that's reading a book, or taking a walk, or watching your favorite show without your partner or kids around. Whatever it is that brings you joy, make time for it. What you feed your soul is just as important as what you feed your body.

Prep Day

Sunday is usually my prep day, and like everything else in my life, I try to keep it simple. I cook all my rice and potatoes for the week, make a big batch of oatmeal for weekday breakfasts, and boil pasta ahead of time, so all I have to do is heat it up and sauce it.

I make sure to have lots of frozen veggies on hand for quick steaming, and I wash and chop all the fresh vegetables that I'll be roasting during the week. That way, all I have to do is reach into my fridge, grab my prepped veggies, throw them in a pan with some seasonings, and roast them! I also make sure I've made a batch of cheese sauce (see page 176) for the week, as well as any other sauces or dressings I think I'll want. You can buy premade sauces instead; just make sure you choose sauces that are oil-free. (If they contain sugar, that's okay in my book— just don't overdo it.)

Make Ahead

1. Cook rice for the week (I steam it in a pressure cooker).

2. Cook potatoes for the week (I steam them in a pressure cooker).

3. Cook oatmeal for the week (I make it in a pressure cooker).

4. Cook pasta for the week (make sure to rinse it well after cooking so it doesn't get hard in the refrigerator during the week).

5. Wash and chop veggies for roasting for the week.

6. Stock up on frozen vegetables.

7. Make cheese sauce and other dressings/sauces you want to have on hand, like ranch and soy ginger sauce (a high-speed blender works best for cheese sauce to get creamy texture).

8. Wash fruit and place it on the kitchen counter or somewhere it's easy to find so you don't reach for something else when you need a snack.

Troubleshooting and Weight Maintenance FAQs

Is it normal to feel full but hungry?

Yes! When you're first transitioning to eating a plant-based diet, your body is adjusting to foods that are naturally lower in calories so you might feel hungry frequently during the initial transition. So if you're hungry, just have some more food.

I feel like I'm eating too much. Is this okay?

Yes! Remember that whole, plant-based foods are low in calories and big in bulk. You need to eat a lot of food to get what you need and still lose weight. I eat HUGE platefuls of food at each meal.

What if I get too full on my nonstarchy veggies and can't eat my starches?

Just reduce the amount of food you are trying to eat, but continue to arrange your plate according to the dilution examples (see pages 13–14).

I feel gassy and bloated. Is this normal?

Yes, it's completely normal. Plants are full of fiber (both soluble and insoluble), and our stomachs need to adjust to digesting it. Drink lots of water and know that it can take up to a few weeks for your body to become accustomed to your new diet.

If you feel uncomfortable, slowly work on adding more veggies into your diet, or talk to your doctor. If you're in severe pain, definitely seek medical attention. Eating a chewable papaya enzyme, like American Health's Original Papaya Enzyme: The "After Meal" Supplement, with each meal can help mitigate gas and bloating as well.

How much weight can I expect to lose every week?

Everyone is different, and the more weight you have to lose, the faster you'll lose it. Conversely, the closer you are to your ideal weight, the slower it will come off. In general, the average amount of weight loss a person can expect in a week is half a pound to a pound. Again, if you have a lot to lose, you may lose more weight more quickly. If you're within a few pounds of where you want to be, it may take longer. Just be consistent in how you eat.

My weight is up three pounds from yesterday—am I doing something wrong?

No. Weight fluctuates daily based on our hormonal cycles, how much sodium we've ingested, and how much water we've had, so aim to weigh yourself only once a week. Do this on the same day every week, first thing in the morning after you have gone to the bathroom and before you've had anything to eat or drink. And do it in your birthday suit (naked).

How many snacks can I have per day?

As many as you need. If you find that you're constantly snacking, though, try to eat more at mealtimes.

My weight loss has stopped, but I still want to lose more—what do I do?

First, make sure you're being really good about low to no fat, avoiding processed foods, and not snacking on anything other than fresh vegetables and whole fresh fruits. If all that looks good, then it might be time to move down in plates. For example, if you have been using the ³⁰/₇₀ plate and have stopped losing weight, then move down to the ⁵⁰/₅₀ plate, and so on. If you're on the ⁷⁰/₃₀ plate (see page 14), and still not losing weight you can preload your meals with a soup or salad to further lower the calorie density of your meals without cutting the volume of food you get to eat.

You can also try eating more raw fruits and vegetables. Try including more salads loaded with raw veggies and even fruits at the start of your meal, and then move on to your ⁵⁰/₅₀ plate for the rest of the meal.

Now that I've lost all the weight I wanted to lose, how do I maintain my weight?

Stick to the ⁵⁰/₅₀ plate, and enjoy treats and some healthy fats from avocado, nuts, and seeds, in moderation. If your weight starts to go up, you know you need to back off on the treats and the fats.

Can I drink any alcohol, or will that keep me from losing weight?

Of course, the choice is yours, but I recommend not drinking alcohol, especially when your goal is to lose weight. You're consuming calories that will not satiate you, and those excess calories from alcohol can really stall weight loss.

Is it normal to have more than three bowel movements a day?

Yes, it is. You're eating a lot of fiber, which adds bulk to your eliminations and increases their frequency. Your body will get used to the fiber, and your number of eliminations may reduce.

Are these recipes family-friendly?

Yes! All the recipes in this book are family-friendly and can be scaled up. My kids love everything from the waffles and pancakes to the enchiladas and egg rolls, and don't even get me started on the desserts! You can adjust these meals to your family's caloric needs by providing extra sauces, dressings, and avocados, as well as increasing portion sizes. On nights when I like to have a burrito bowl, my husband and kids eat theirs with tortillas, extra cheese sauce, and avocado, and top everything with cashew sour cream. This helps them take in the extra calories they need. They also eat larger portions of starches like rice and potatoes than I do (since I'm not a growing teenager!).

Master Pantry List

Keep these items on hand for easy and quick prep. There's nothing like needing an ingredient to stall even the best intentions to prep for the week.

- Baking powder
- Black salt (kala namak)
- Buffalo wing sauce (I like Frank's RedHot in mild)
- Chili flakes
- Chili paste, oil-free (like sambal oelek)
- Chili powder
- Cocoa nibs or dairy-free chocolate chips
- Coconut extract (optional)
- Cumin seeds
- Curry powder
- Dijon mustard
- Distilled white vinegar
- Dried dill (optional)
- Dried moong dal (split mung beans)
- Dried oregano
- Dried parsley
- Dried thyme
- Garam masala
- Garlic powder
- Garlic salt
- Ground black pepper
- Ground coriander
- Ground turmeric
- Hot sauce (optional)
- Instant yeast
- Liquid smoke
- Minced jarred ginger
- Minced jarred garlic
- Mustard, Dijon
- Mustard, yellow
- Nori sheets (i.e., seaweed sheets)
- Nutritional yeast
- Oat flour
- Onion powder
- Powdered peanut butter (such as PB2)
- Pure maple syrup
- Pure vanilla extract
- Red curry paste
- Rolled oats
- Saffron strands (optional)
- Seasoned rice vinegar
- Sesame seeds
- Smoked paprika
- Soy sauce (low-sodium)
- Sugar, unrefined or coconut
- Vegan bouillon cubes (I like Edward & Sons Not-Chick'n)
- Vegan hoisin sauce
- White rice
- Whole wheat flour (or all-purpose gluten-free flour)
- Worcestershire sauce (vegan)

Sample 28-Day Meal Plan

This sample meal plan is between 1,500 and 1,800 calories per day, not including snacks and desserts. You'll have to decide if this amount of food is right for you, based on your size and how active you are. If you have a lot of weight to lose, you may need more calories in the beginning, so eat according to your appetite while being sure to always use the ⁵⁰⁄₅₀ plate or one of the other plate options (see pages 13–14). If you're still hungry, look to the snack section (see chapter 4).

Keep in mind that this meal plan is just an example! If this is too much variety and cooking for you, make your own meal plan, and make it simple and repetitive. For simplicity's sake, I like to make my lunch for the next day from dinner's leftovers, so feel free to double the recipes so you have extra. Make this lifestyle work for *you*!

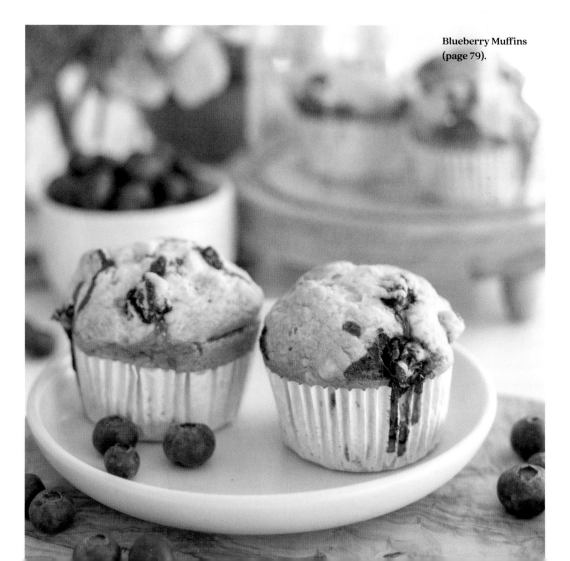

Blueberry Muffins (page 79).

Week 1

MONDAY	**BREAKFAST** Tofu Scramble with whole-grain toast, 2 large oranges, sliced Calories: 518	**LUNCH** Eggless Egg Salad Sammy, House Salad Calories: 500	**DINNER** Loaded Baked Potato Calories: 529	Total Daily Calories: 1,547
TUESDAY	**BREAKFAST** Sunrise Smoothie, toast spread with 2 tablespoons mashed banana (optional) Calories: 519	**LUNCH** Baked Potato leftovers Calories: 529	**DINNER** Tortilla Lime Soup, South-west Salad (without beans, rice, and avocado) Calories: 564	Total Daily Calories: 1,612
WEDNESDAY	**BREAKFAST** Buff Avocado Toast, 2 cups sliced strawberries Calories: 505	**LUNCH** Tortilla Lime Soup leftovers, Southwest Salad (without beans, rice, and avocado) Calories: 564	**DINNER** Chili Cheese Fries, House Salad Calories: 682	Total Daily Calories: 1,751
THURSDAY	**BREAKFAST** Berry Cereal Calories: 562 cals	**LUNCH** Buffalo Chickpea Salad Wrap, House Salad Calories: 493	**DINNER** Persian Rice and Chickpea Bowl, Roasted Brussels Sprouts Calories: 509	Total Daily Calories: 1,564
FRIDAY	**BREAKFAST** Apple Streusel Oats; 1 large orange, sliced Calories: 482	**LUNCH** Persian Rice and Chickpea Bowl leftovers, Roasted Brussels Sprouts Calories: 509	**DINNER** 7 Egg Rolls Calories: 572 cals	Total Daily Calories: 1,563
SATURDAY	**BREAKFAST** Vanilla Cinnamon French Toast, 2 cups berries Calories: 498	**LUNCH** Egg Roll leftovers Calories: 572	**DINNER** Nachos, Steamed Asparagus Calories: 571	Total Daily Calories: 1,641
SUNDAY	**BREAKFAST** Biscuits and Gravy, Garlic Roasted Zucchini and Onion Calories: 465	**LUNCH** Nachos, Steamed Asparagus Calories: 571	**DINNER** Macaroni and Cheese, Caesar Salad Calories: 534	Total Daily Calories: 1,570

Week 2

	BREAKFAST	LUNCH	DINNER	
MONDAY	Smoky Southern Potatoes with Gravy, Roasted Brussels Sprouts and Mushroom Mix Calories: 536	Curry Hummus Sammy, House Salad Calories: 463	Cheesy Broccoli Rice Casserole Calories: 558	Total Daily Calories: 1,557
TUESDAY	Green Goodness Smoothie, 1 slice of toasted sprouted whole-grain bread spread with 2 tablespoons mashed banana (optional) Calories: 469	Cheesy Broccoli Rice Casserole leftovers Calories: 558	Sweet Potato with Curry-Roasted Chickpeas, Turmeric-Roasted Cauliflower Calories: 617	Total Daily Calories: 1,644
WEDNESDAY	3 Blueberry Muffins, 1¼ cups grapes Calories: 513	Philly "Cheesesteak" Spuds Calories: 546	Thai Coconut Curry with 1¼ cups steamed rice Calories: 577	Total Daily Calories: 1,636
THURSDAY	Peach Cobbler Oats, 2 additional large peaches or plums, pitted and sliced Calories: 519	Thai Coconut Curry with 1¼ cups steamed rice Calories: 577	Easy Enchiladas, Garlic Roasted Zucchini and Onion Calories: 638	Total Daily Calories: 1,734
FRIDAY	3 Banana Muffins, 2 sliced apples with cinnamon Calories: 509	Spring Roll Bowl Calories: 632	Crunchy Tostada Wrap, Southwest Salad (without the rice, beans, and avocado) Calories: 654	Total Daily Calories: 1,795
SATURDAY	Pumpkin Spice Waffles, 1 cup sliced strawberries Calories: 518	Crunchy Tostada Wrap leftovers, Taco Salad (without the rice, beans, and avocado) Calories: 654	Asian Lettuce Wraps with 1 cup steamed rice Calories: 523	Total Daily Calories: 1,695
SUNDAY	Vegetable Omelet, 2 cups sliced strawberries Calories: 428	Asian Lettuce Wrap leftovers with 1 cup steamed rice Calories: 523	Creamy Poblano Soup, Steamed Broccoli with Cheese Sauce Calories: 588	Total Daily Calories: 1,539

Week 3

MONDAY	**BREAKFAST** Breakfast Burrito; 1 orange, sliced Calories: 488	**LUNCH** Creamy Poblano Soup leftovers, Steamed Broccoli with Cheese Sauce Calories: 588	**DINNER** Chickpea Curry with 1 cup steamed rice, Turmeric-Roasted Cauliflower Calories: 600	Total Daily Calories: 1,676
TUESDAY	**BREAKFAST** Buff Avocado Toast; 1 apple, sliced Calories: 478	**LUNCH** Chickpea Curry leftovers with 1 cup steamed rice, Turmeric-Roasted Cauliflower Calories: 600	**DINNER** Chinese Vegetables and Rice Calories: 475	Total Daily Calories: 1,553
WEDNESDAY	**BREAKFAST** 3 Banana Muffins, 2 cups berries Calories: 489	**LUNCH** Chinese Rice and Vegetables leftovers Calories: 475	**DINNER** Easy Creamed Potatoes, Steamed Asparagus Calories: 543	Total Daily Calories: 1,507
THURSDAY	**BREAKFAST** Berry Cereal Calories: 562	**LUNCH** Easy Creamed Potatoes leftovers, Steamed Asparagus Calories: 543	**DINNER** Shiitake Rice with Bok Choy and Thai Peanut Sauce Calories: 576	Total Daily Calories: 1,681
FRIDAY	**BREAKFAST** Berry Citrus Smoothie Bowl Calories: 541	**LUNCH** Shiitake Rice with Bok Choy and Thai Peanut Sauce leftovers Calories: 576	**DINNER** Buffalo Cauliflower Wing Salad Calories: 531	Total Daily Calories: 1,648
SATURDAY	**BREAKFAST** Cinnamon Roll Biscuits, 2 cups sliced strawberries Calories: 478	**LUNCH** Buffalo Cauliflower Wing Salad leftovers Calories: 531	**DINNER** 3 "Crab" Rangoon, 3¼ Egg Rolls, Eggless Egg Drop Soup Calories: 587	Total Daily Calories: 1,596
SUNDAY	**BREAKFAST** Vegetable Omelet; 1 orange, sliced Calories: 414	**LUNCH** Spring Ramen Soup Calories: 560	**DINNER** Chickpea "Chicken" Salad Sammy, House Salad Calories: 590	Total Daily Calories: 1,564

Week 4

MONDAY	**BREAKFAST** Buff Avocado Toast, 1 sliced apple Calories: 478	**LUNCH** Chickpea "Chicken" Salad Sammy, House Salad Calories: 593	**DINNER** Chickpea Curry with 1 cup steamed rice, Turmeric-Roasted Cauliflower Calories: 604	Total Daily Calories: 1,675
TUESDAY	**BREAKFAST** Breakfast Berry Cereal Calories: 562	**LUNCH** Buffalo Chickpea Salad Wrap, House Salad Calories: 495	**DINNER** Asian Lettuce Wraps with 1 cup steamed rice Calories: 467	Total Daily Calories: 1,524
WEDNESDAY	**BREAKFAST** Green Goodness Smoothie, 1 slice sprouted whole-grain bread spread with 2 tablespoons mashed banana (optional) Calories: 569	**LUNCH** Persian Rice and Chickpea Bowl, Caesar Salad Calories: 546	**DINNER** Easy Enchiladas Calories: 578	Total Daily Calories: 1,693
THURSDAY	**BREAKFAST** Vegetable Omelet; 1 large orange, sliced Calories: 438	**LUNCH** Burrito Bowl, 1 cup grapes Calories: 542	**DINNER** Easy Creamed Potatoes, Roasted Brussels Sprouts with Maple Mustard Dressing Calories: 623	Total Daily Calories: 1,603
FRIDAY	**BREAKFAST** Breakfast Burrito, 1 cup berries Calories: 502	**LUNCH** Warm White Bean and Potato Salad Calories: 535	**DINNER** Pizza Calories: 558	Total Daily Calories: 1,595
SATURDAY	**BREAKFAST** Blueberry Vanilla Pancakes, 1 cup berries Calories: 576	**LUNCH** Chickpea "Chicken" Salad Sammy, House Salad Calories: 593	**DINNER** Buffalo Cauliflower Wing Salad Calories: 531	Total Daily Calories: 1,700
SUNDAY	**BREAKFAST** Vanilla Waffles Calories: 448	**LUNCH** Philly "Cheesesteak" Spuds Calories: 546	**DINNER** Crunchy Tostada Wrap, Garlic Roasted Zucchini and Onion Calories: 579	Total Daily Calories: 1,573

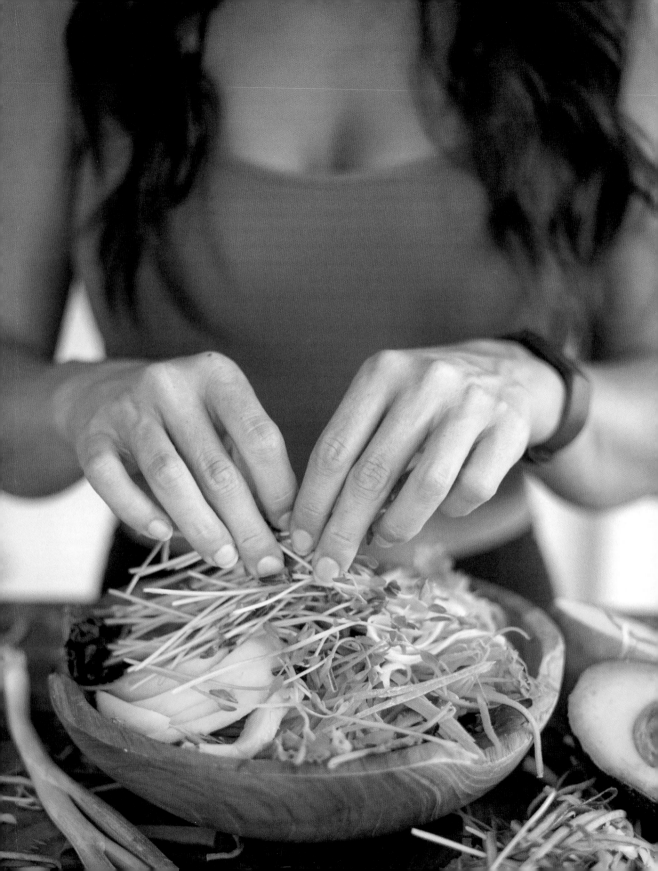

PART

3

The
Recipes

CHAPTER 1

Breakfast

Blueberry Vanilla Pancakes

MAKES
10
PANCAKES

Blueberry vanilla pancakes—need I say more? These are deliciously moist and can be made with fresh or frozen berries. I do use a little bit of maple syrup, but fresh or thawed blueberries are a great topping, too. Or try an all-natural low-calorie sugar-free syrup, like the one by Lakanto.

1¼ cups whole wheat flour, oat flour, or gluten-free flour

2 teaspoons baking powder

½ teaspoon sea salt

2 tablespoons unrefined sugar, such as coconut sugar or pure maple syrup (optional)

1 teaspoon pure vanilla extract

½ cup fresh or frozen blueberries, plus more for serving

Avocado oil cooking spray (optional)

2 tablespoons pure maple syrup, for serving (optional)

1. In a medium bowl, stir together the flour, baking powder, and salt. Add the sugar (if using), the vanilla, and 1¼ cups water. Stir until combined. Gently fold in the blueberries.

2. Heat a nonstick griddle or pan over medium-high heat. Lightly spray the pan with avocado oil if yours likes to stick. Working in batches, use a ¼-cup measuring cup to scoop the batter onto the griddle, leaving a few inches between each pancake. Cook for 2 minutes, or until the bottom of each pancake begins to brown. Flip the pancakes and cook for 2 minutes more, until cooked through and golden brown on the second side. Transfer the finished pancakes to a plate and repeat with the remaining batter. Enjoy with more blueberries and a drizzle of maple syrup, if desired.

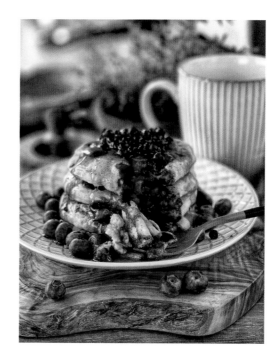

NUTRITION INFORMATION
SERVING SIZE: 5 pancakes with 1 tablespoon maple syrup   **CALORIES:** 384   **PROTEIN:** 10 g   **CARBS:** 78 g   **FAT:** 2 g

Vegetable Omelet

This plant-based omelet is so delicious and full of wholesome and filling ingredients, such as moong dal, also known as split mung beans, which get soaked overnight and are rich in protein. I fill the omelets with spinach, tomatoes, and mushrooms and top them with cheese sauce and hot sauce. If you're new to a vegan diet, I promise that you really won't miss eggs. The moong dal mixture is wonderfully light and airy, and with all the vegetables and sauce, these omelets are satisfying. They're a welcome change from the usually heavy and high-calorie egg omelets we often make at home, and certainly from the omelets usually served in restaurants.

½ cup dried moong dal (split mung beans), soaked overnight

¼ cup white rice flour

¾ teaspoon black salt (kala namak; see Note opposite)

¾ teaspoon baking powder

½ teaspoon garlic powder or minced fresh garlic

½ teaspoon onion powder

¼ teaspoon ground turmeric (optional, for color)

2 cups sliced white mushrooms

¼ cup minced yellow onion

Avocado oil cooking spray (optional)

1 cup packed fresh baby spinach leaves

¼ cup diced tomatoes

¼ cup Cheese Sauce (page 176), warmed

Salsa, hot sauce, or ketchup, for serving (optional)

1. Drain and rinse the moong dal well under cold running water. In a blender, combine the moong dal, rice flour, black salt, baking powder, garlic powder, onion powder, and turmeric, if using. Add ¾ cup water and blend until smooth. Set aside.

2. In a large nonstick skillet, cook the mushrooms and onions over medium-high heat, adding a splash of water to help them soften, until vegetables are tender, 3 to 5 minutes. Transfer the mushrooms and onion to a medium bowl and set aside.

3. Wipe out the pan and return it to the heat. If your pan likes to stick, lightly coat it with avocado oil. Using a ⅓-cup measuring cup, add one scoop of the egg mixture to the pan. Swirl to coat the bottom of the pan and cook for 2 to 4 minutes, until the omelet is no longer runny on the top and the bottom is beginning to set. Flip the omelet and cook for 2 to 4 minutes more, until set and golden brown on the bottom. Transfer the omelet to a plate and repeat with the remaining egg mixture, making 5 omelets total.

4. Top each omelet with the mushroom-onion mixture, spinach, and tomatoes. Drizzle the vegetables with cheese sauce, then fold the omelets in half and drizzle the tops with more sauce. Enjoy with salsa, hot sauce, or ketchup.

NUTRITION INFORMATION
SERVING SIZE: 2 omelets   CALORIES: 332   PROTEIN: 16 g   CARBS: 54 g   FAT: 5 g

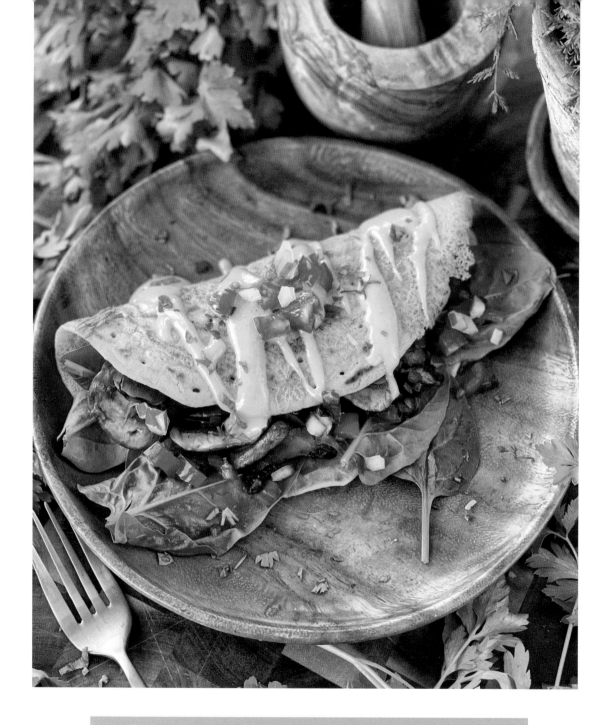

NOTE: I like using black salt, also known as kala namak, for this recipe. It has a slightly eggy flavor that makes this dish taste like it's actually made with eggs. If you prefer, you could use sea salt instead.

Breakfast Burrito

MAKES
2
BURRITOS

Who doesn't love a good breakfast burrito? They are bright and delicious, and always filling. I love these for two reasons: One, because they use the simple omelet mixture from page 52, and two, because it is so easy to batch prep these babies! If you have leftover omelet mixture or just a little time to do some week-ahead planning, make these burritos and store them in the freezer (they freeze amazingly well), then pop them straight from the freezer into the microwave or toaster oven when you need a quick breakfast or snack.

utes, or try toasting them in a nonstick pan until the tortilla turns golden, 1 to 2 minutes per side.

> NOTE: I like Olé Mexican Foods Xtreme Wellness tortillas and wraps because they contain almost no fat. You could also use gluten-free tortillas. Or skip the tortillas entirely and turn these into breakfast bowls by adding 1 to 2 cooked medium potatoes instead.

2 (10-inch) tortillas (see Note)

2 Vegetable Omelets (page 52), chopped into bite-size pieces

2 cups spring greens

½ cup cooked or canned pinto beans (drained and rinsed, if canned)

2 Roma (plum) tomatoes, diced

½ small avocado, sliced (optional)

½ cup Cheese Sauce (page 176), warmed

¼ cup plus 2 tablespoons salsa, store-bought or homemade

Your favorite hot sauce (optional)

Lay the tortillas on a work surface. Top each evenly with the omelet, greens, beans, tomatoes, avocado (if using), cheese sauce, salsa, and hot sauce, if desired. Carefully roll them up and serve. Or, if you like, heat the burritos in the microwave for 1½ min-

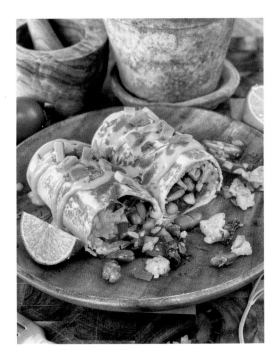

NUTRITION INFORMATION
SERVING SIZE: 1 burrito (without avocado)   **CALORIES:** 416   **PROTEIN:** 21 g   **CARBS:** 52 g   **FAT:** 11 g

Smoky Southern Potatoes with Gravy

SERVES
2

When I'm in the mood for a savory breakfast, I always think, Potatoes and Gravy. There are really only two components to this dish—the potatoes, and the mushroom gravy—and both can be made ahead of time and reheated.

NOTE: Feel free to use leftover cooked potatoes instead of roasting raw ones. You'll need about 3 cups diced cooked potatoes. Season and then bake at 350°F for 10 minutes to crisp them up again before using.

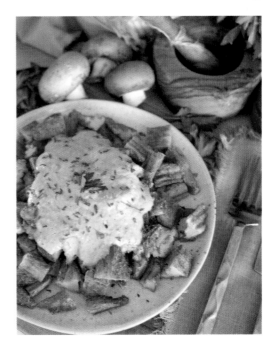

4 medium Yukon Gold potatoes, cut into 1-inch pieces (see Note)

½ teaspoon garlic salt, or more if you like things garlicky

½ teaspoon smoked paprika

Freshly ground black pepper

2 cups Mushroom Gravy (page 190), warmed

1. Preheat the oven to 425°F. Arrange the potatoes on a baking sheet and sprinkle them with the garlic salt, paprika, and pepper. Toss to coat the potatoes well. Bake for 20 to 30 minutes, until the potatoes are golden, crisp, and tender.

2. Divide the potatoes between two plates and top them with the gravy, then serve.

NUTRITION INFORMATION
SERVING SIZE: 1 serving   **CALORIES:** 471   **PROTEIN:** 14 g   **CARBS:** 88 g   **FAT:** 3 g

Buff Avocado Toast

SERVES

2

Avocado toast is one of those meals that's comforting yet light and nourishing at the same time. Here the fat-free refried beans also bring fiber and protein to the meal and make it an even more filling and nutritious breakfast. Try topping this with a little Everything Bagel Seasoning for some extra flavor and texture!

1 small avocado

4 slices sprouted whole-grain or gluten-free bread (see Note), toasted

1 cup fat-free refried beans, homemade or store-bought, warmed

1 cup sprouts or microgreens

¼ cup Cheese Sauce (page 176), warmed (optional)

Your favorite hot sauce (optional)

1. In a small bowl, use a fork to mash the avocado.

2. Spread the avocado over the toast. Top with the beans and sprouts, and finish with a drizzle of cheese sauce and/or hot sauce, if desired.

NOTE: My favorite bread is Ezekiel 4:9 sprouted whole-grain bread; for a gluten-free option, I'll use Outside the Breadbox vegan oat bread—feel free to use what you like.

NUTRITION INFORMATION
SERVING SIZE: 1 serving, including Cheese Sauce   **CALORIES:** 399   **PROTEIN:** 17 g   **CARBS:** 40 g   **FAT:** 13 g

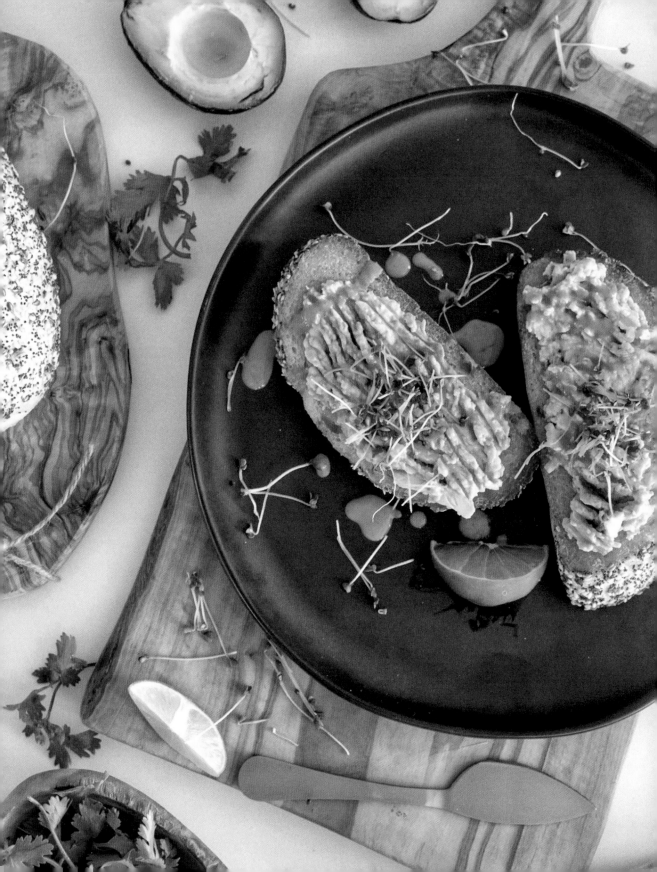

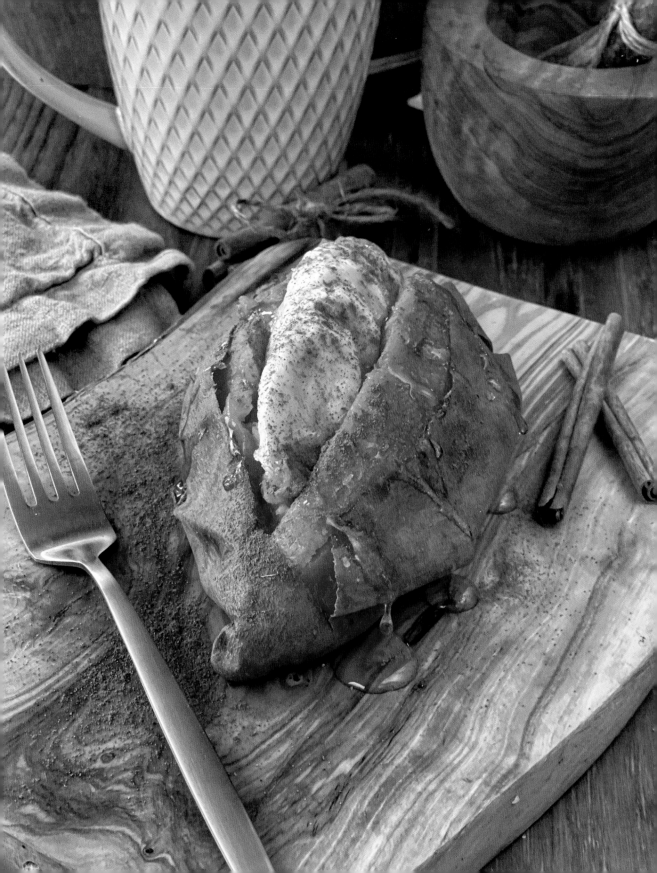

Maple Pecan Sweet Potatoes

SERVES
2

Sweet potatoes are one of the most nutritious foods. They're full of vitamins such as A and C and minerals including sleep-promoting magnesium. Just 3.5 ounces will give you 47 percent of your daily vitamin C requirement! They will keep you full and satisfied and can be batch prepped ahead of time and reheated when you're ready to use them (they'll keep for 3 to 4 days in the refrigerator). The light drizzle of maple syrup and sprinkle of pecans really go a long way in taking these simple, nutritious root vegetables over the top.

2 large sweet potatoes, scrubbed, rinsed, and dried
2 small bananas, sliced
2 tablespoons chopped pecans
2 teaspoons pure maple syrup
Dash of ground cinnamon

1. Preheat the oven to 400°F. Place the sweet potatoes on a baking sheet and bake for 35 to 45 minutes, until you can easily pierce them with a knife.

2. Divide the potatoes between two plates, split them lengthwise, and top with the bananas, pecans, maple syrup, and cinnamon. Enjoy warm.

NUTRITION INFORMATION
SERVING SIZE: 1 serving   **CALORIES:** 498   **PROTEIN:** 8 g   **CARBS:** 93 g   **FAT:** 5 g

Biscuits and Gravy

Biscuits and gravy was always a weekend comfort food in my house when I was growing up. When I switched to a plant-based diet, I knew I needed to find a way to make this super-satisfying favorite dish in a healthy, cleaned-up way so I could continue to enjoy it while on my weight loss journey.

---

2 cups whole wheat flour or gluten-free flour (I like Bob's Red Mill Gluten Free 1-to-1 Baking Flour; see Note)

2 teaspoons baking powder

½ teaspoon sea salt

2 cups Mushroom Gravy (page 190), warmed

Thyme, for garnish

---

1. Preheat the oven to 375°F. Line a baking sheet with parchment paper or a silicone baking mat.

2. In a medium bowl, mix together the flour, baking powder, and salt. While stirring, slowly add 1½ cups water and stir until just combined. You want the batter to be slightly lumpy.

3. Use a spoon to drop the batter onto the prepared baking sheet in 7 even portions. Bake for 15 to 20 minutes, until the biscuits are starting to brown.

4. Place two biscuits on each plate (you'll have three left over for snacking!). Spoon the gravy over the biscuits, sprinkle with herbs, and enjoy.

> **NOTE:** While I recommend using whole wheat or gluten-free flour to make this recipe as healthy as possible, you can use all-purpose flour. You'll just need to adjust the water to 1¼ cups.

NUTRITION INFORMATION
SERVING SIZE: 2 biscuits with 1 cup gravy   **CALORIES:** 346   **PROTEIN:** 15 g   **CARBS:** 58 g   **FAT:** 4.3 g

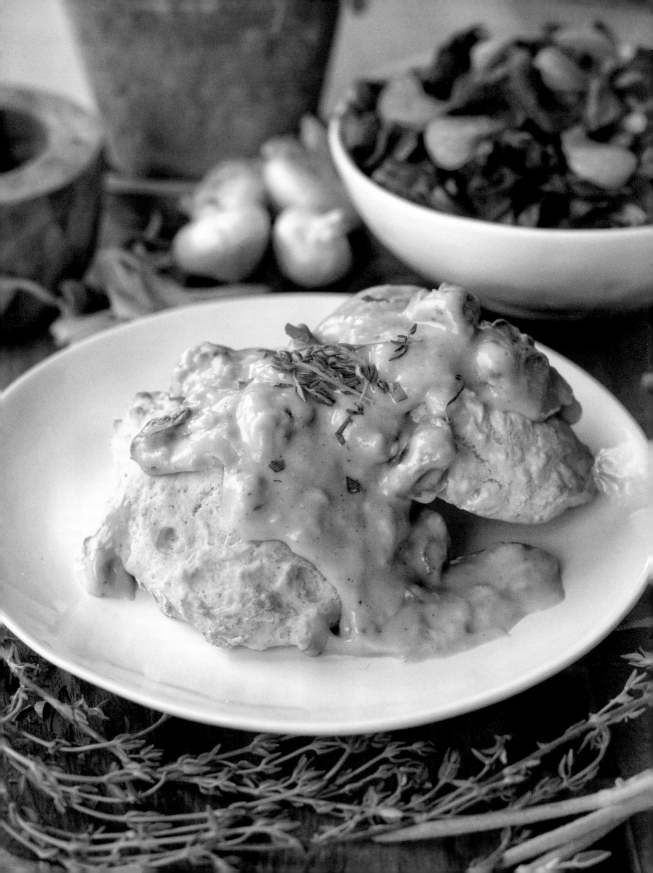

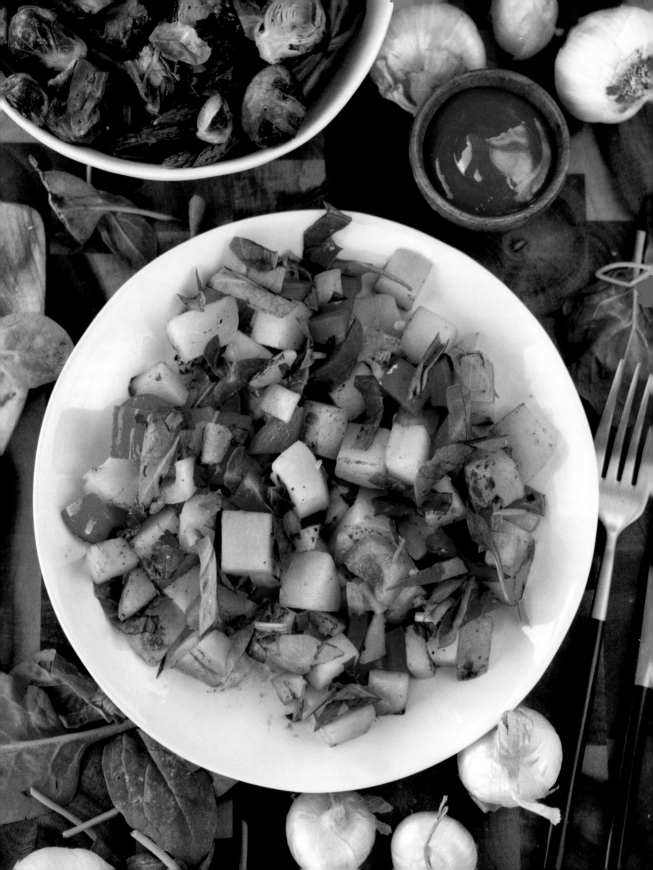

Breakfast Hash

SERVES
2

There always seems to be a day at the end of the week where I have a little bit of bell pepper and onion and just enough spinach sitting around to make it worth adding them to a dish. Mushrooms bring a hearty, meaty flavor to this hash, and roasting all those leftover bits together makes a quick and tasty breakfast. If you're pressed for time, you can lightly spray a nonstick skillet with avocado oil and brown the hash up on the stovetop instead of waiting for it to roast in the oven or air fryer.

**4 medium Yukon Gold potatoes,
cut into 1-inch pieces**

1 cup diced red bell pepper

½ cup diced yellow onion

**½ teaspoon garlic salt, or more
if you like things garlicky**

Ground black pepper

2 tablespoons vegetable broth (optional)

2 cups chopped fresh spinach leaves

**Ketchup and/or your favorite hot sauce,
for serving (optional)**

1. Preheat the oven 425°F. On a baking sheet, combine the potatoes, bell pepper, and onion. Season with the garlic salt, black pepper, and broth (if using) and toss to mix well. Roast for 20 to 30 minutes, until the vegetables are browned and tender.

2. Divide the vegetables between two plates and mix in the spinach. Enjoy with ketchup and/or hot sauce.

NOTE: Feel free to use leftover cooked potatoes instead of roasting raw ones. You'll need about 4 cups diced cooked potatoes. When roasting your vegetables, I give you the option of tossing them with a little vegetable broth to help keep them from sticking to the pan—a handy oil-free trick!

NUTRITION INFORMATION
SERVING SIZE: 1 serving   **CALORIES:** 403   **PROTEIN:** 10 g   **CARBS:** 80 g   **FAT:** 1 g

Breakfast Berry Cereal

SERVES
2

If you were an '80s kid like me, you probably ate lots of boxed cereal. When our family would try to "eat better," we would have granola with milk instead. But now we all know that granola has even more fat and calories than many processed cereals! This berry cereal combines a big bowl of berries with some of my oil-free granola and almond milk to make a crunchy and satisfying breakfast.

2 cups hulled strawberries
1 cup blueberries
1 cup blackberries or raspberries
1 small banana, sliced
2 peaches, pitted and diced
1½ cups Weight Loss–Friendly Granola (page 206)
2 cups unsweetened almond milk
(I like Almond Breeze; see Note)

In each cereal bowl, combine half the berries, banana, peaches, and granola. Top with the milk and enjoy.

NOTE: Instead of almond milk, you can use any plant-based milk with around 30 calories per cup.

NUTRITION INFORMATION
SERVING SIZE: 1 serving   **CALORIES:** 562   **PROTEIN:** 13 g   **CARBS:** 101 g   **FAT:** 7 g

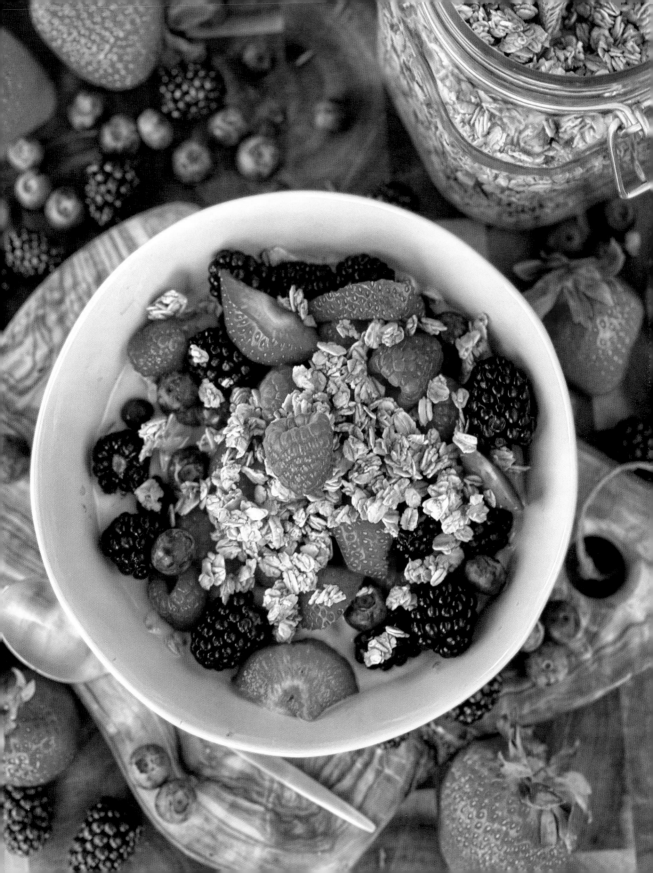

Vanilla Waffles

I've always been intimidated by making waffles, but then I realized I could throw everything into a blender to make the batter! Now waffles are a part of our regular rotation, and the flavor options are endless. Experiment with lemon extract and poppy seeds, or add maple extract and cinnamon for a comforting waffle with the flavors of fall. I love to use anise extract around the holidays because it reminds me of the pizzelles my mom used to make growing up. I make a big batch of these and freeze them, so that anyone in the family can pop a few in the toaster for a quick breakfast!

2 cups rolled oats
2 overripe medium bananas
2 teaspoons pure vanilla extract
1 teaspoon baking powder
Pinch of sea salt
Avocado oil cooking spray (optional)
2 tablespoons pure maple syrup (optional)

1. Preheat a waffle iron. In a blender, combine the oats, bananas, vanilla, baking powder, and salt. Add 1½ cups water and blend until smooth.

2. Lightly spray the waffle iron with avocado oil, if yours likes to stick. Pour ⅓ cup of the batter into the waffle iron and cook until the waffle is golden and no longer sticking to the plates, 8 to 10 minutes. Transfer the cooked waffle to a plate and repeat with the remaining batter. Serve with maple syrup, if desired.

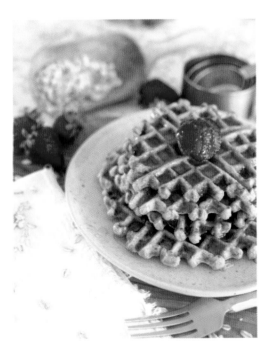

NUTRITION INFORMATION
SERVING SIZE: 5 waffles with 1 tablespoon maple syrup   **CALORIES:** 460   **PROTEIN:** 12 g   **CARBS:** 81 g   **FAT:** 6 g

Cinnamon Roll Oats

These oats remind me of the oats my mom used to make me when I was a kid. The simple, sweet flavor of a little brown sugar and cinnamon is always comforting, and the crunch from the heart-healthy walnuts adds a delicious texture.

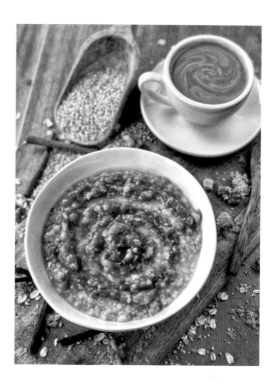

2 small bananas

1 teaspoon pure vanilla extract

1 teaspoon ground cinnamon

1 cup rolled oats, cooked according to the package instructions

2 tablespoons chopped walnuts

2 tablespoons packed brown sugar

In a medium bowl, use a fork to mash the bananas with the vanilla and cinnamon. Stir in the cooked oats. Divide the mixture between two bowls, then top with the walnuts and brown sugar. Enjoy warm.

NUTRITION INFORMATION
SERVING SIZE: 1 serving   **CALORIES:** 353   **PROTEIN:** 8 g   **CARBS:** 58 g   **FAT:** 8 g

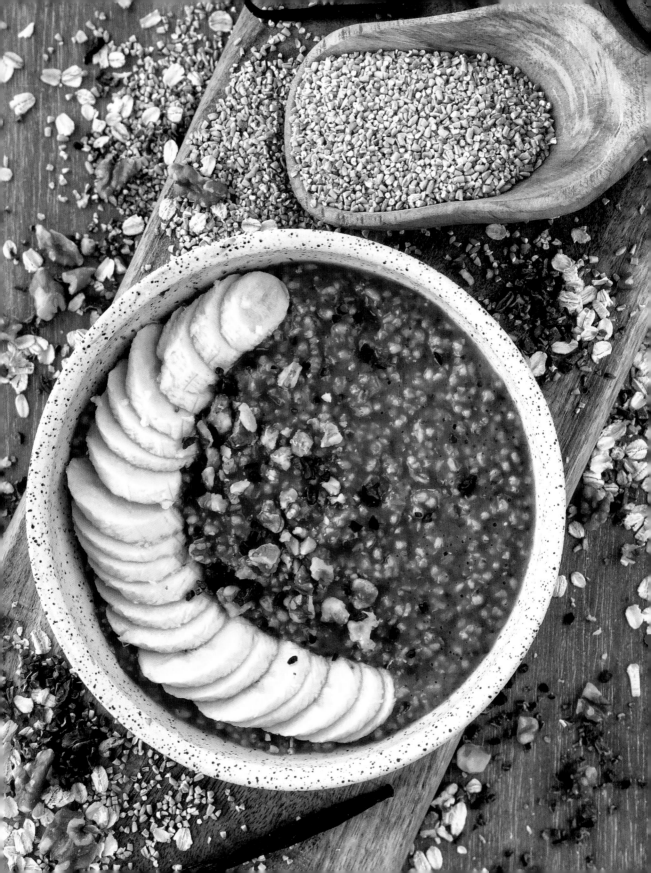

Chocolate Crunch Oats

SERVES
2

Oatmeal seems to be something that people either love or hate. It's definitely polarizing in my house! I happen to love oatmeal—I love how creamy and warm and filling it is—but my husband and kids do not. They hate it. But it's amazing how a little chocolate can persuade the naysayers. This oatmeal is sweet and decadent-seeming, and sometimes I even make it for dessert.

1 cup rolled oats, cooked according to the package instructions

2 small bananas, sliced

2 tablespoons unsweetened cocoa powder

2 tablespoons chopped walnuts

2 tablespoons pure maple syrup

1 teaspoon pure vanilla extract

In a medium bowl, combine the cooked oats, bananas, cocoa powder, walnuts, maple syrup, and vanilla. Divide between two individual serving bowls and enjoy warm.

NUTRITION INFORMATION
SERVING SIZE: 1 serving   **CALORIES:** 361   **PROTEIN:** 9 g   **CARBS:** 59 g   **FAT:** 9 g

Peach Cobbler Oats

I always look forward to summer, when the fresh peaches from our orchard ripen. A fresh-picked peach, so succulent and sweet that you have to eat it outside or over the sink so as not to get the juices everywhere, can be a dessert all by itself. But adding it to my oatmeal with the same ingredients that make a peach cobbler so fantastic—banana, cinnamon, vanilla, and maple syrup—make this both simple and wholesome. Have a peach cobbler for breakfast!

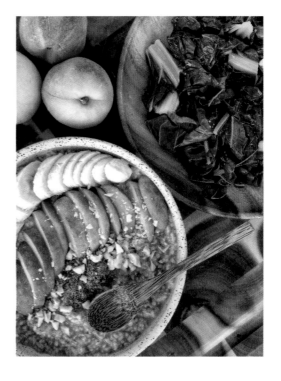

1 cup rolled oats, cooked according to the package instructions

2 tablespoons pure maple syrup

1 teaspoon pure vanilla extract

Pinch of ground cinnamon

2 small bananas, sliced

2 peaches, pitted and diced

In a medium bowl, combine the oats, maple syrup, vanilla, and cinnamon. Divide between two individual serving bowls and top with bananas and peaches.

NUTRITION INFORMATION
SERVING SIZE: 1 serving   **CALORIES:** 388   **PROTEIN:** 9 g   **CARBS:** 75 g   **FAT:** 4 g

Apple Streusel Oats

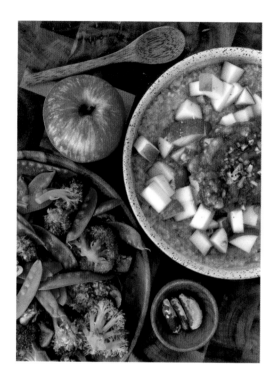

Apple pie for breakfast? Yes, please! The warm chunks of apple and delicate hints of vanilla and cinnamon in this breakfast treat are topped with the delicious crunch of omega-3 rich walnuts. This is a crowd-pleasing breakfast. It's filling before a big day, and comforting on a cold or rainy morning. Try this with Honeycrisp apples; they give this oatmeal an almost cider-like taste.

2 small bananas

1 teaspoon pure vanilla extract

½ teaspoon ground cinnamon

1 cup rolled oats, cooked according to the package instructions

2 medium Honeycrisp apples, cored and diced

2 tablespoons chopped walnuts

In a medium bowl, use a fork to mash the bananas with the vanilla and cinnamon. Stir in the oats and apples. Divide between two individual serving bowls, top with the walnuts, and enjoy warm.

NUTRITION INFORMATION
SERVING SIZE: 1 serving   **CALORIES:** 392   **PROTEIN:** 8 g   **CARBS:** 64 g   **FAT:** 8 g

Pumpkin Spice Waffles

I'm one of those people who brings out the fall decorations and the pumpkin spice as soon as September hits! For these waffles, just throw all the ingredients into your blender and whirl up the batter. Make sure to lightly spray your waffle iron with avocado oil, and keep the lid of the iron down longer than you think you should. If the waffles are coming apart, you need to let them cook a little longer.

---

2 cups rolled oats

2 ripe medium bananas

½ cup canned pure pumpkin puree

2 teaspoons pure vanilla extract

1 teaspoon pumpkin pie spice

Avocado oil cooking spray

2 tablespoons pure maple syrup (optional), or fruit

---

1. Preheat a waffle iron. In a blender, combine the oats, bananas, pumpkin puree, vanilla, and pumpkin pie spice. Add 1½ cups water and blend until smooth.

2. Lightly spray the waffle iron with avocado oil. Pour ⅓ cup of the batter into the waffle iron and cook until the waffle is golden and no longer sticking to the plates, 5 to 8 minutes. Transfer the cooked waffle to a plate and repeat with the remaining batter. Serve with maple syrup, if desired, or fruit.

NUTRITION INFORMATION
SERVING SIZE: 7 waffles with 1 tablespoon maple syrup   **CALORIES:** 481   **PROTEIN:** 12 g   **CARBS:** 84 g   **FAT:** 6 g

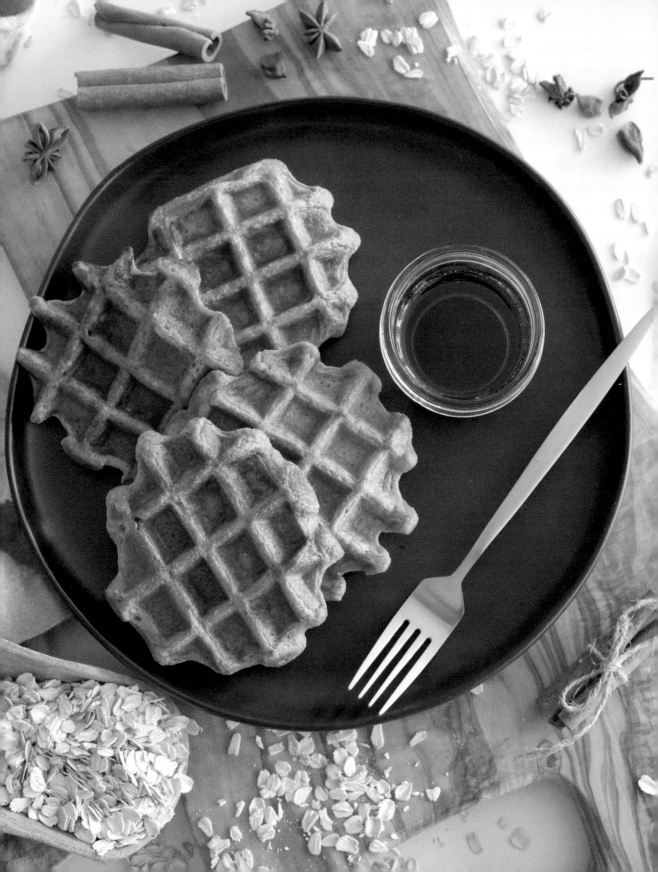

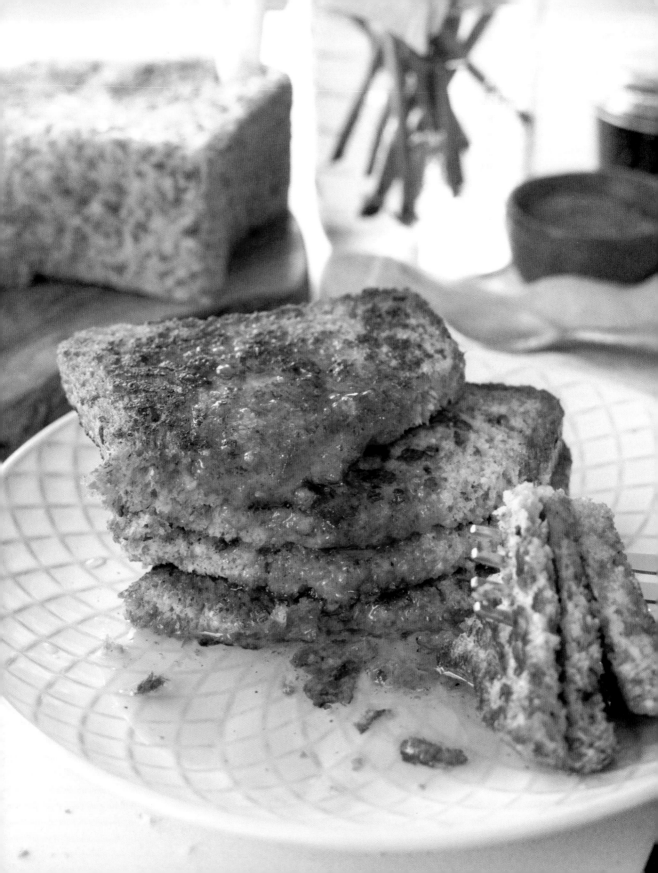

Vanilla Cinnamon French Toast

When we were growing up, my siblings and I looked forward to French toast every Sunday, and the same is now true for my family. When we made the transition to a plant-based diet, my children were concerned about losing their Sunday French toast, but I like a challenge ... and it turns out you can still make great French toast without eggs. The trick is to use a hearty, denser bread like a sprouted whole-grain loaf. I like the one Ezekiel 4:9 makes; when you squeeze it, you can tell it's sturdy, not soft, so it won't turn to mush in your pan.

Avocado oil cooking spray (optional)

1½ cups plant-based milk

2 teaspoons pure vanilla extract

½ teaspoon ground cinnamon

8 slices sprouted whole-grain bread or gluten-free bread (see Note)

2 tablespoons pure maple syrup, or ½ cup mashed banana

1. Heat a nonstick griddle or skillet over medium heat. Lightly coat with avocado oil, if yours likes to stick.

2. In a shallow bowl, stir together the milk, vanilla, and cinnamon. Dip each slice of bread into the batter until well coated. Arrange the toast on the griddle, working in batches if necessary. Cook for 3 minutes, or until golden brown on the bottom. Flip and cook for 3 minutes more, or until golden brown on the second side. Transfer to a plate and repeat with the remaining bread. Serve with the maple syrup or mashed banana.

NUTRITION INFORMATION
SERVING SIZE: 4 pieces of toast with 1 tablespoon maple syrup or ¼ cup mashed banana   **CALORIES:** 410   **PROTEIN:** 17 g
CARBS: 64 g   **FAT:** 4 g

⬤ Tofu Scramble

I'm admittedly not crazy about tofu. (There, I said it.) But I found that when I prepared it in a "scramble" with all my favorite vegetables, I absolutely love it! The tofu soaks up the flavor of the seasonings and the veggies and has an egglike texture. My husband and kids devour this, too. Try adding some cheese sauce (see page 176) to the top and some hot sauce for a little extra kick.

---

16 ounces white mushrooms, chopped

1 red bell pepper, diced

1 small yellow onion, diced

1 tablespoon vegetable broth or water

1 (16-ounce) package extra-firm tofu, drained and crumbled

Pinch of ground turmeric

Sea salt and freshly ground black pepper

---

1. In a large nonstick pan, combine the mushrooms, bell pepper, onion, and broth.

2. Cook over medium-high heat, stirring occasionally, until the vegetables have begun to brown, about 5 minutes.

3. Add the tofu and turmeric, and season with salt and black pepper. Cook until the tofu is just heated through, 1 to 2 minutes more. Taste and adjust the seasoning with more salt and black pepper, if needed. Serve warm.

NUTRITION INFORMATION

SERVING SIZE: 1 serving **CALORIES:** 252 **PROTEIN:** 30 g **CARBS:** 8 g **FAT:** 13 g

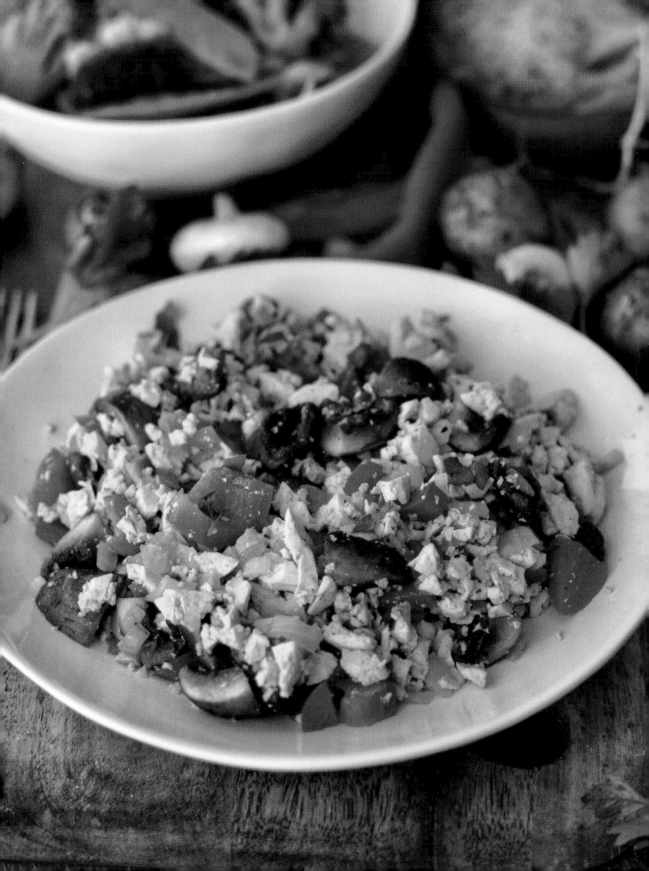

Banana Muffins

My best friend Nicole makes the most wonderful banana bread, and she never uses a recipe! She just throws ingredients into a bowl, mixes the batter, pours it into a pan, and bakes it. Her banana bread is delicious every single time. When I was trying to develop a vegan banana bread recipe, it failed every time, but then I found success making the batter into muffins! The batter sets up better when it's baked into muffins, as it doesn't dry out. Little pro tip: If you have kiddos who need a little bit of sweet to soothe their junk food cravings, just add a few chocolate chips to the batter—they'll gobble up the muffins and feel well indulged!

1½ cups whole wheat flour or oat flour (see Note)

¼ cup unrefined sugar or coconut sugar

1 tablespoon powdered vegan egg replacer or ground flaxseed

1 teaspoon baking powder

¼ teaspoon baking soda

⅛ teaspoon sea salt

2 overripe medium bananas, mashed

1 teaspoon pure vanilla extract

1. Preheat the oven to 375°F. Line 8 cups of a standard 12-cup muffin tin with paper liners.

2. In a medium bowl, stir together the flour, sugar, egg replacer, baking powder, baking soda, and salt. Add the bananas, vanilla, and 1 cup water. Stir until just combined; do not overmix.

3. Divide the batter evenly among the prepared muffin cups. Bake for 22 to 24 minutes, until a cake tester inserted into the center of a muffin comes out clean. Enjoy warm, or let the muffins cool completely, then store them in an airtight container at room temperature for up to 3 days or freeze for up to 1 month.

NOTE: To make this recipe gluten-free, use oat flour instead of whole wheat.

NUTRITION INFORMATION
SERVING SIZE: 3 muffins   **CALORIES:** 375   **PROTEIN:** 10 g   **CARBS:** 76 g   **FAT:** 2 g

Blueberry Muffins

MAKES
8
MUFFINS

In Estes Park, Colorado, there's a little coffee shop that I love called Kind Coffee. Whenever I'm in town for a hiking trip, I stop there for a blueberry muffin. They're full of sweet blueberries, and the muffin itself is never too sugary. I decided I needed to make my own cleaned-up plant-based version, and I think they're pretty good: moist and full of blueberry flavor. If you're gluten-free, you can swap out the wheat flour for gluten-free oat flour and the muffins will still come out great. I think using fresh blueberries makes them even more delicious, and I love baking them at the height of blueberry season, but frozen berries work just fine, too.

1½ cups whole wheat flour or oat flour

¼ cup unrefined sugar or coconut sugar

1 tablespoon powdered vegan egg replacer or ground flaxseed

1 teaspoon baking powder

¼ teaspoon baking soda

⅛ teaspoon sea salt

¼ cup unsweetened applesauce or mashed banana

1 teaspoon pure vanilla extract

1 cup fresh or frozen blueberries

1. Preheat the oven to 375°F. Line 8 wells of a muffin tin with paper liners.

2. In a medium bowl, stir together the flour, sugar, egg replacer, baking powder, baking soda, and salt. Add the applesauce (or banana, if using), vanilla, and 1 cup water. Stir until just combined; do not overmix. Gently fold in the blueberries.

3. Add ¼ cup of the batter to each of the prepared muffin cups. Bake for 18 to 20 minutes, until a cake tester inserted into the center of a muffin comes out clean. Enjoy warm, or let the muffins cool completely, then store them in an airtight container at room temperature for up to 3 days or freeze them for up to 1 month.

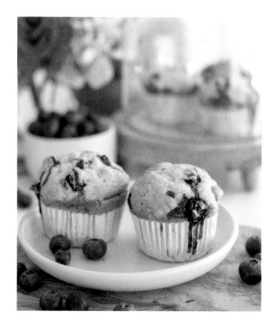

NUTRITION INFORMATION
SERVING SIZE: 3 muffins   **CALORIES:** 363   **PROTEIN:** 9 g   **CARBS:** 72 g   **FAT:** 2 g

Sunrise Smoothie

Sometimes you just need a super-quick breakfast, and that's where smoothies come in. They're the perfect choice for a breakfast on the go. With fresh orange juice and strawberries, this drink is citrusy and blends perfectly with the bananas. If bananas aren't your thing, try substituting fresh or frozen mango for that added creaminess.

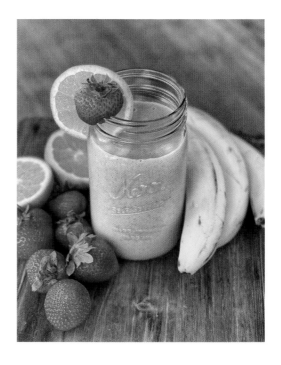

2 cups fresh or frozen strawberries

2 medium bananas

½ cup plain, unsweetened plant-based milk (see Note)

Juice of 1 orange

½ teaspoon pure vanilla extract

In a blender, combine the strawberries, bananas, milk, orange juice, and vanilla. Blend until smooth.

NOTE: I like Almond Breeze almond milk, but use any plain, unsweetened plant-based milk you like with around 30 calories per cup.

NUTRITION INFORMATION

SERVING SIZE: 1 smoothie   CALORIES: 421   PROTEIN: 6 g   CARBS: 87 g   FAT: 3 g

Green Goodness Smoothie

Green smoothies are one of my favorite ways to get in an extra serving or two of greens, which are the most nutrient-dense food groups on the planet, and we could all benefit from more of them! If you want to add another little powerhouse to this smoothie, try blending in a piece of peeled fresh ginger. It will amp up the flavor with a nice kick!

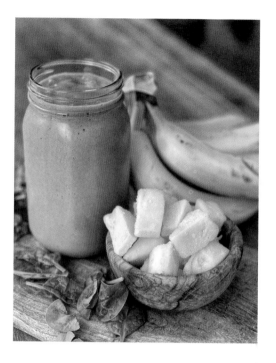

2 very ripe large bananas
2 cups packed fresh spinach leaves
1 cup frozen pineapple (see Note)

In a blender, combine the bananas, spinach, pineapple, and 1 cup water, then blend until smooth.

NOTE: If you only have fresh pineapple, add a handful of ice before blending to make this smoothie even creamier.

NUTRITION INFORMATION
SERVING SIZE: 1 smoothie   **CALORIES:** 326   **PROTEIN:** 6 g   **CARBS:** 72 g   **FAT:** 1 g

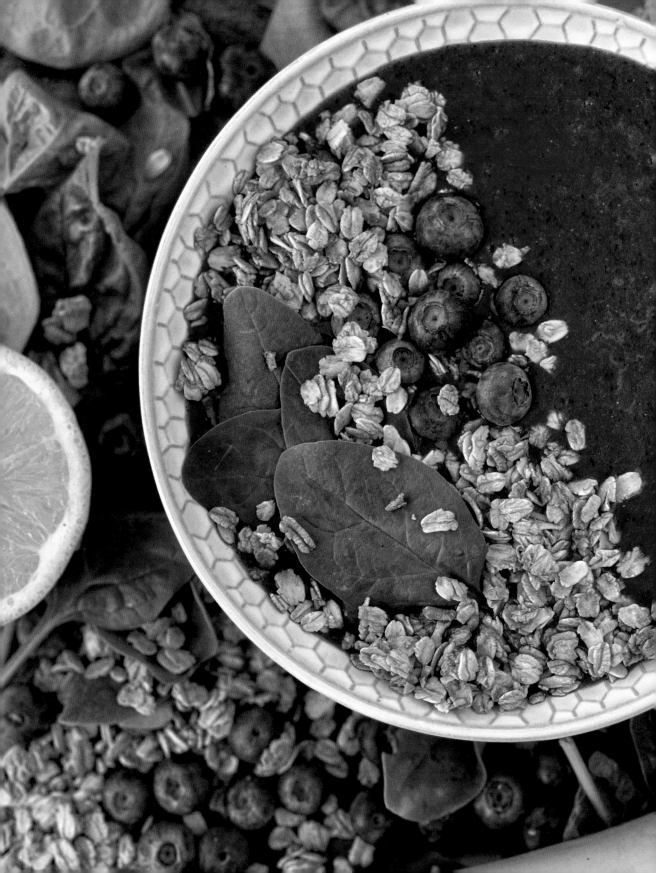

Berry Citrus Smoothie Bowl

MAKES
1
32-OUNCE
SMOOTHIE

This guy is an antioxidant powerhouse! Full of antioxidant-rich blueberries, spinach, and orange juice, it will hydrate you and your skin. If you want some crunch and texture, top it off with a little granola (see page 206) and some berries for an easy smoothie bowl.

2 medium bananas

2 cups frozen blueberries

2 cups packed fresh spinach leaves

Juice of 1 orange

½ cup fresh berries (optional)

½ cup Weight Loss–Friendly Granola (page 206; optional)

1. In a blender, combine the bananas, blueberries, spinach, and orange juice. Add ½ cup water and blend until smooth.

2. Pour into a bowl and top with Weight Loss–Friendly Granola (page 206) and ½ cup fresh berries, if you like.

NUTRITION INFORMATION
SERVING SIZE: 1 smoothie bowl with ½ cup granola and ½ cup berries   **CALORIES:** 609   **PROTEIN:** 11 g   **CARBS:** 121 g   **FAT:** 5 g

CHAPTER 2

Lunch and Dinner

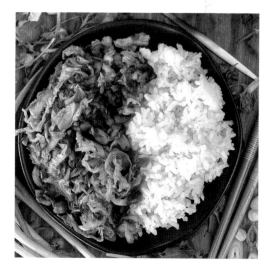 Chinese Rice and Vegetables

I love Asian-inspired meals. This combination is not only incredibly nutritious and low in calories but also rich in flavor and filling, with the combination of meaty mushrooms, crunchy cabbage, and rice. Beyond steaming the rice and chopping the vegetables, there's almost no prep to this. The small amount of toasted sesame oil I include makes the dish, in my opinion. I eat this on repeat throughout the week, and I highly recommend serving it with Eggless Egg Drop Soup (page 141).

2 cups finely shredded napa cabbage

8 ounces baby bella (cremini) mushrooms, chopped

½ cup diced yellow onion

3 tablespoons low-sodium soy sauce

¼ cup fresh cilantro leaves, chopped (optional)

1 green onion, white and green parts thinly sliced

¼ teaspoon toasted sesame oil (optional; see Note)

Pinch of chili flakes (optional)

2 tablespoons chopped roasted unsalted cashews (optional; see Note)

4 cups white or brown rice, cooked

1. In a large pot or sauté pan with a fitted lid, combine the cabbage, mushrooms, onion, and soy sauce. Cover and cook over medium-high heat until the vegetables release their liquid, about 3 minutes. Remove the lid and cook until the vegetables are tender and most of the liquid has evaporated, 5 to 10 minutes. Remove the pan from the heat.

2. Stir in the cilantro (if using), green onion, and, if desired, the sesame oil and chili flakes. Top with the nuts, if you like, and serve with the steamed rice.

> **NOTE:** The toasted sesame oil and chopped roasted cashews are optional, but add flavor and texture here. If you choose to include the oil, add 10 calories and 1 gram of fat to the nutritional totals; if you include the nuts, add 98 calories and 8 grams of fat.

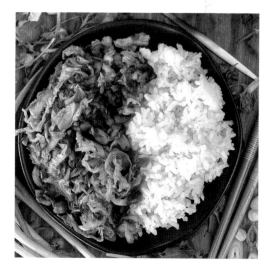

NUTRITION INFORMATION

SERVING SIZE: 1 cup vegetable mix and 2 cups steamed rice   **CALORIES:** 475   **PROTEIN:** 14 g   **CARBS:** 95 g   **FAT:** 2 g

Sweet Potato with Curry-Roasted Chickpeas

SERVES

1

This simple combination of sweet potato topped with curry-roasted chickpeas and arugula and drizzled with my vegan Caesar dressing is absolutely delicious—the flavors just pop in your mouth! I roast the chickpeas, wash the arugula (or buy it prewashed), and cook the sweet potatoes early in the week, then keep everything in the fridge so I can throw together this simple but delicious dish any time I need a quick and satisfying meal.

1 medium sweet potato

1 cup packed arugula

½ cup Curry-Roasted Chickpeas (page 205)

¼ cup Caesar Dressing (page 175)

1. Preheat the oven to 425°F. Prick the top of the potato with a fork, place on a baking sheet, and roast for 40 to 50 minutes, until you can easily pierce it with a knife.

2. Slice the potato in half lengthwise and top each half evenly with the arugula, chickpeas, and dressing.

NUTRITION INFORMATION

SERVING SIZE: 1 serving   **CALORIES:** 478   **PROTEIN:** 17 g   **CARBS:** 71 g   **FAT:** 9 g

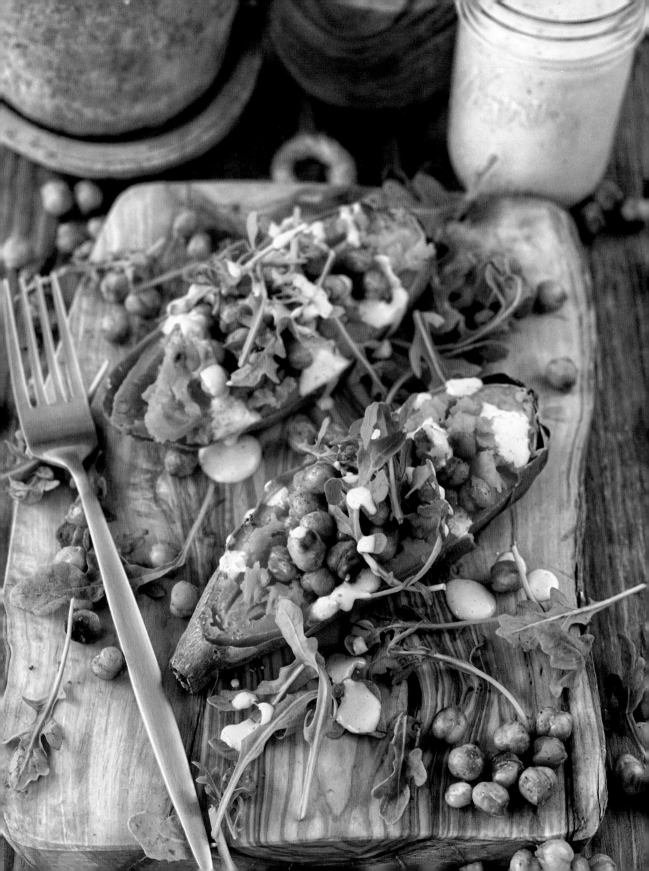

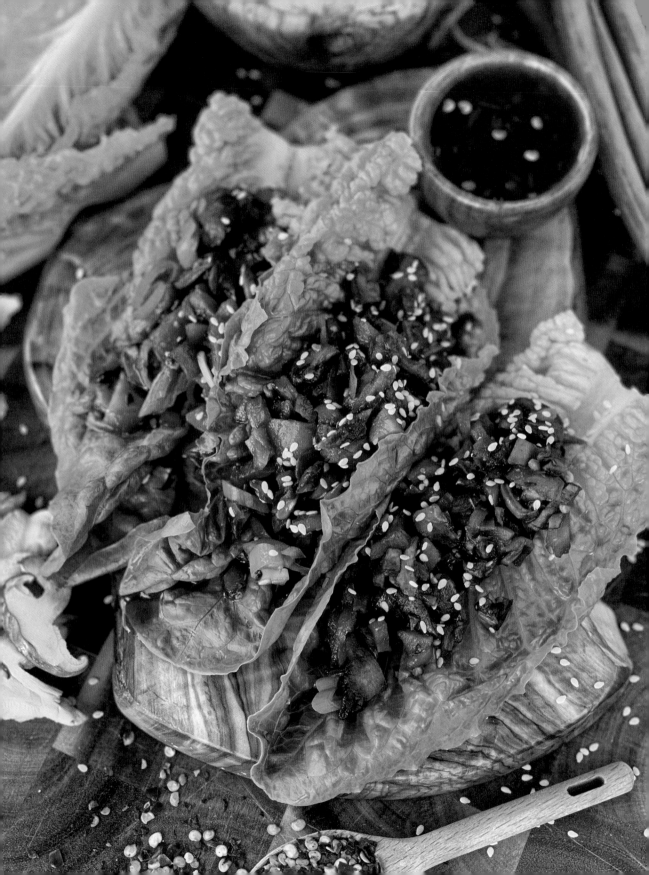

Asian Lettuce Wraps

SERVES
2

I know I'm hardly the first person to discover lettuce wraps, but I think they're truly genius. They're less caloric than sandwiches and, I think, more satisfying because they're fresh and crunchy. These lettuce wraps are my mom's favorite, and she asks me to make them for her every time I visit. She loves the light, tangy flavor, and the heartiness that the mushrooms add. Even my little one (who swears she doesn't like mushrooms) loves this!

16 ounces white mushrooms (see Note), chopped

2 (8-ounce) cans sliced water chestnuts, drained

½ cup minced yellow onion

1 green onion, white and green parts sliced

1 tablespoon minced garlic

¼ cup low-sodium soy sauce

¼ cup hoisin sauce (I like Wok Mei gluten-free hoisin)

¼ cup seasoned rice vinegar

2 tablespoons pure maple syrup

2 teaspoons oil-free chili paste (I like sambal oelek; optional)

10 romaine lettuce leaves

4 cups white or brown rice, cooked

1. In a large sauté pan, combine the mushrooms, water chestnuts, yellow onion, green onion, and garlic. Cook over medium-high heat, stirring occasionally, until the vegetables are soft, about 10 minutes.

2. Meanwhile, in a medium bowl, stir together the soy sauce, hoisin, vinegar, maple syrup, and chili paste (if using).

3. When the vegetables are soft, add the sauce to the pan and cook for 2 to 3 minutes, until the sauce clings to the vegetables. Remove the pan from the heat.

4. To serve, wrap the filling in the romaine leaves and enjoy with a side of steamed rice, if desired.

NOTE: If you don't like mushrooms, try eggplant or zucchini instead. They sauté beautifully.

NUTRITION INFORMATION
SERVING SIZE: 1 serving (with 1 cup rice)   **CALORIES:** 541   **PROTEIN:** 18 g   **CARBS:** 106 g   **FAT:** 4 g

Chickpea Curry

SERVES
4

I could eat curry in some form every night of the week. The key to bringing out the strongest flavors is to cook your spices first in the tomato puree, so don't skip that step!

---

1 (15-ounce) can crushed tomatoes

½ medium yellow onion, chopped

1 tablespoon minced garlic

1 teaspoon minced fresh ginger, or ¼ teaspoon ground ginger

⅛ teaspoon cumin seeds

1 teaspoon curry powder

1 teaspoon ground coriander

1 teaspoon garam masala

½ teaspoon sea salt, plus more as needed

1 (29-ounce) can or 2 (12.5-ounce) cans chickpeas, drained and rinsed

⅓ cup plain, unsweetened plant-based milk

Chopped fresh cilantro leaves, for garnish

4 cups white or brown rice, cooked, for serving (optional)

---

1. In a blender, combine the tomatoes, onion, garlic, and ginger. Blend until smooth and set aside.

2. In a large sauté pan, toast the cumin seeds over medium-high heat until fragrant and just beginning to brown, 1 to 2 minutes. Add the blended tomato mixture, the toasted cumin seeds, curry powder, garam masala, and salt. Bring the mixture to a simmer and then cook, stirring occasionally, for 5 to 10 minutes, until it has reduced and thickened slightly.

3. Add the chickpeas and milk and remove the pan from the heat. Taste and adjust the seasoning with more salt, if needed. Garnish with cilantro and serve with rice, if desired.

> NOTE: This is a super-flavorful dish, and the garam masala and the yellow curry meld together perfectly in the tomato sauce with the garlic and ginger. This will freeze well, and any leftovers will last all week.

NUTRITION INFORMATION
SERVING SIZE: 1 serving (with 1 cup rice) **CALORIES:** 425 **PROTEIN:** 16 g **CARBS:** 71 g **FAT:** 5 g

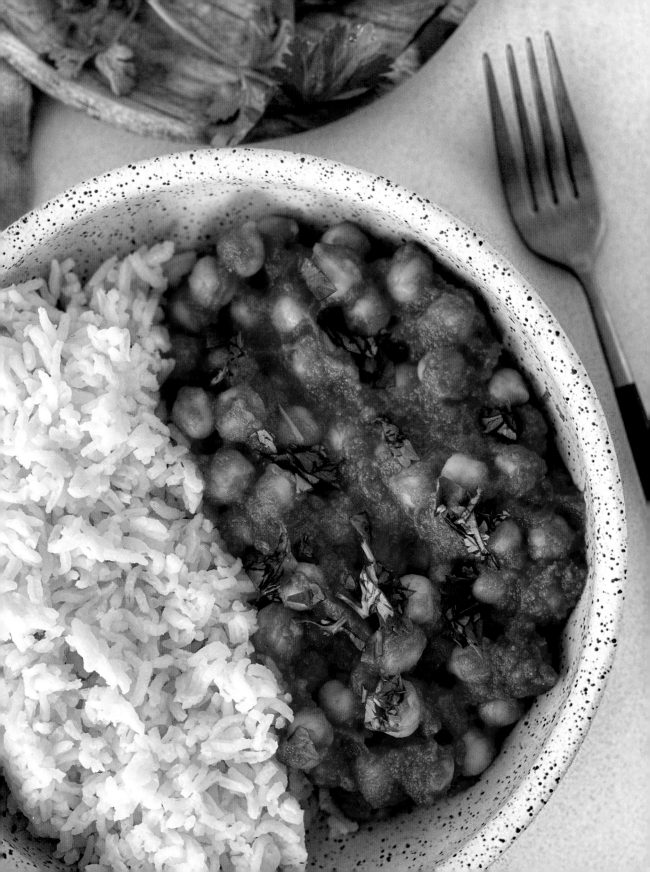

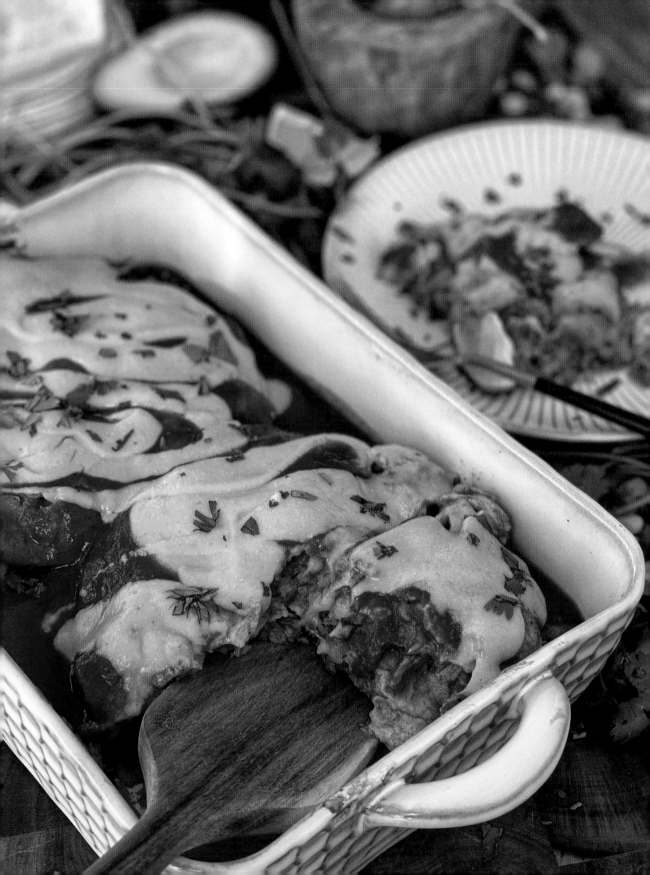

Easy Enchiladas

SERVES
2

I grew up on enchilada casserole, so when I switched to a plant-based diet, I wanted to find a way to remake this favorite dish from my childhood. This is truly a simple and easy-to-pull-together dish, especially if you already have some cooked potatoes hanging out in your fridge! You can make double or triple the recipe and freeze it or keep it in the fridge all week to enjoy. This is one of my family's favorite weeknight meals.

2 medium Yukon Gold or russet potatoes, cooked

1 cup fat-free refried beans,
store-bought or homemade

½ cup salsa, store-bought or homemade

½ cup canned corn kernels, drained

½ cup fresh cilantro leaves

2 tablespoons fresh lime juice

Sea salt

6 (6-inch) corn tortillas

1½ cups fat-free enchilada sauce
(I like Hatch organic red enchilada sauce)

½ cup Cheese Sauce (page 176), warmed

1 cup chopped lettuce

1. Preheat the oven to 400°F. In a medium bowl, use a fork to mash the cooked potatoes. Mix in the refried beans, salsa, corn, cilantro, and lime juice. Taste and adjust the seasoning with salt, if needed.

2. Spread a spoonful of the enchilada sauce over the bottom of an 8 x 12-inch oven-safe baking dish. Lay 3 tortillas over the sauce to cover the bottom of the dish. Spread half the potato filling over the tortillas, followed by half the remaining enchilada sauce. Repeat with the remaining tortillas, following by the remaining filling, and finally the remaining sauce.

3. Cover the baking dish with aluminum foil and bake for 20 minutes, until the sauce is bubbling and the enchiladas are warmed through. Top with the cheese sauce, sprinkle with the lettuce, and serve.

NUTRITION INFORMATION
SERVING SIZE: 1 serving   **CALORIES:** 545   **PROTEIN:** 18 g   **CARBS:** 90 g   **FAT:** 5 g

Smokehouse Steak Fries

SERVES
2

If you have cooked potatoes ready to go in your fridge, these steak fries are especially easy to make. I actually think having precooked potatoes make for a crispier fry. That said, if you're using cooked potatoes, make sure they're completely cooled, even cold from the fridge; otherwise, when you go to shake them up with the seasonings, they'll fall apart. If you're having a hard time warming up to the idea of oil-free potatoes, don't be afraid to give these a light spray of cooking oil to help them crisp up. As you get more accustomed to cooking without oil, you may find you're okay with omitting it. (But I would rather you use a little spray oil and eat nutritious food than not use it and miss out on this delicious dish.)

4 medium Yukon Gold potatoes
2 teaspoons garlic powder
1 teaspoon onion powder
½ teaspoon smoked paprika
½ teaspoon sea salt
Ketchup (optional)

1. Preheat the oven to 425°F. Line a baking sheet with parchment paper.

2. Place the potatoes in a small pot and add enough cold water just to cover them. Bring the water to a boil over medium-high heat, then reduce the heat to maintain a simmer. Cook the potatoes until they can be easily pierced with a fork, 15 to 20 minutes. (Alternatively, steam the potatoes on the stovetop or in the microwave for 10 to 15 minutes.) Remove and let cool.

3. When the potatoes are cool enough to handle, slice them into thick wedges and place them in a food storage container with a lid. Sprinkle over the garlic powder, onion powder, paprika, and salt. Cover the container and give everything a vigorous shake so the potatoes are evenly coated and a little roughed up, which helps them crisp in the oven.

4. Arrange the potatoes on the prepared baking sheet and bake for 15 to 20 minutes, until golden and crisp. Serve immediately, with ketchup if desired.

NUTRITION INFORMATION
SERVING SIZE: 1 serving   **CALORIES:** 319   **PROTEIN:** 7 g   **CARBS:** 65 g   **FAT:** 0 g

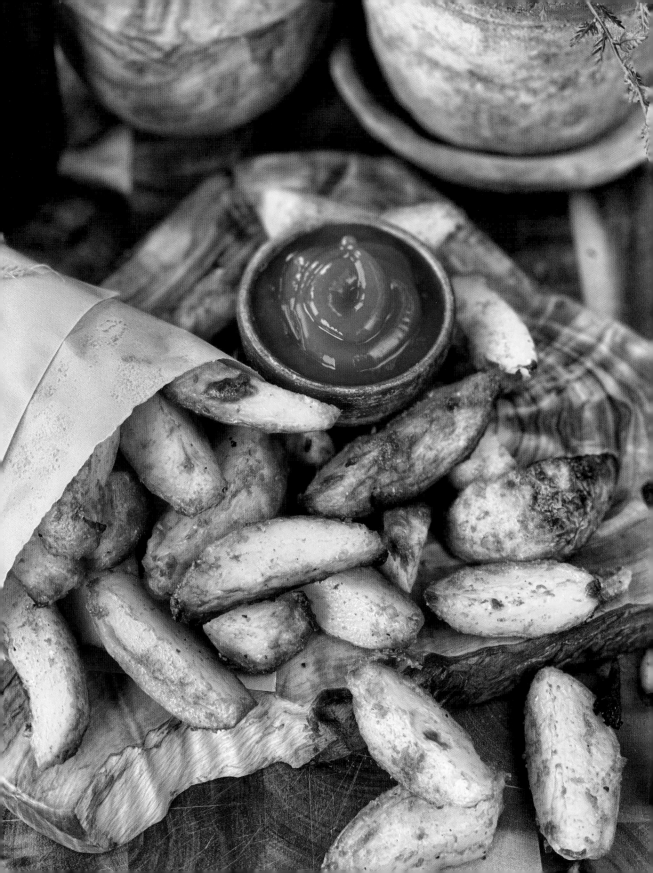

Persian Rice and Chickpea Bowl

SERVES
2

My babysitter growing up was named Farah. How I loved Farah. She was a kind and gentle Iranian woman who was always making us the most amazing Persian food. My mom finally stopped packing our lunches because we only ever wanted to eat Farah's cooking. Her specialty of specialties, which I absolutely loved, was this amazing saffron rice bowl, topped with simple, fresh ingredients and a delicious yogurt sauce. This is my take on the lunch that Farah used to make for me most days. I like to add fresh tomatoes and parsley or cilantro and green onions for garnish, but you can add diced cucumber or fresh green beans as well.

2 cups white or brown rice
Pinch of saffron (optional)
1 cup canned chickpeas, drained and rinsed
1 cup chopped Roma (plum) tomatoes
1 green onion, white and green parts chopped
1 tablespoon chopped fresh parsley leaves
Garlic salt
½ cup Cashew Ranch Dressing (page 181)

1. Cook the rice according to the package instructions, adding the saffron to the water when you add the rice, if desired.

2. Transfer the cooked rice to a large bowl and add the chickpeas, tomatoes, green onion, and parsley. Taste and season with garlic salt. Toss with the ranch dressing just before serving.

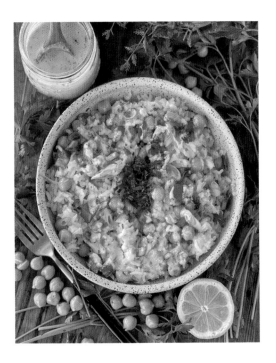

NUTRITION INFORMATION
SERVING SIZE: 1 serving   **CALORIES:** 385   **PROTEIN:** 13 g   **CARBS:** 59 g   **FAT:** 8 g

Easy Creamed Potatoes

SERVES

2

It's no secret that I love comfort food! And one of the best experiences on my journey has been developing easy ways to remake my favorite foods into healthy, weight loss–promoting versions of themselves. I think these potatoes are one of my greatest hits. They're creamy and savory, and they couldn't be easier to pull together. The trick is finding a good thick plant milk. I like Westsoy soy milk and the almond milk from Three Trees Organics.

2 large Yukon Gold or russet potatoes, thinly sliced

2 cups thick, plain, unsweetened plant-based milk (see headnote)

2 teaspoons garlic powder

1 teaspoon onion powder

1 teaspoon chopped fresh rosemary

½ teaspoon fresh thyme leaves

1½ teaspoons sea salt

Pinch of ground black pepper

1. Preheat the oven to 375°F. Arrange the potato slices in a single layer over the bottom of an 8 x 6-inch oven-safe baking dish.

2. In a small bowl, mix together the milk, garlic powder, onion powder, rosemary, thyme, salt, and pepper. Pour the mixture over the potatoes.

3. Cover the baking dish with aluminum foil and bake for 30 minutes, or until the potatoes are tender, and serve hot.

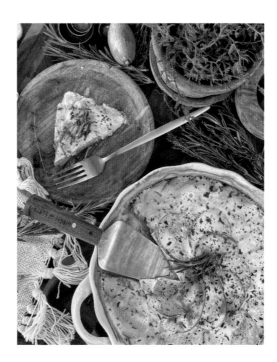

NUTRITION INFORMATION
SERVING SIZE: 1 serving   **CALORIES:** 420   **PROTEIN:** 11 g   **CARBS:** 66 g   **FAT:** 10 g

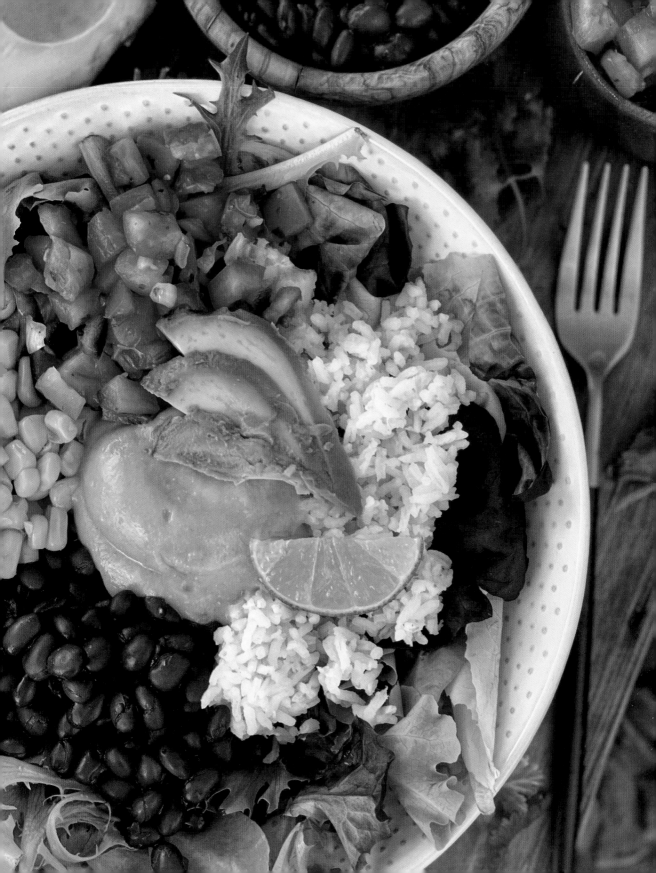

Burrito Bowl

Who doesn't love a good burrito bowl? I find that they're one of the easiest meals to throw together—it just takes a tiny bit of prep. The payoff (and again, the prep is so worth it) is a super-filling dish that's full of nutritious ingredients. A good salsa and my cheese sauce add tons of flavor to any combination in your burrito bowl!

4 cups spring greens or lettuce of your choice

4 cups white or brown rice, cooked

1 cup canned pinto or black beans, drained and rinsed

½ cup fresh or canned corn kernels, drained

½ cup salsa, store-bought or homemade

2 tablespoons minced red onion

Garlic salt

½ small avocado, sliced (optional)

½ cup Cheese Sauce (page 176), warmed

Fresh lime juice, for serving

Chopped fresh cilantro leaves, for garnish (optional)

1. In two wide bowls, create a bed of the greens, dividing them evenly.

2. Top with the rice, then the beans, corn, and salsa. Sprinkle the onion and a good pinch of garlic salt over the top. Top with the avocado (if using), drizzle with the cheese sauce, and squeeze over a bit of lime juice. Sprinkle with cilantro, if desired, and serve.

NUTRITION INFORMATION
SERVING SIZE: 1 serving (with ¼ small avocado)   **CALORIES:** 491   **PROTEIN:** 17 g   **CARBS:** 89 g   **FAT:** 7 g

Warm White Bean and Potato Salad

SERVES
2

This dish came together when my daughter brought in a basket full of our homegrown potatoes, red onions, and fresh arugula. We quickly seasoned and roasted the small potatoes and then tossed them with the arugula. We decided to add white beans and a little red onion and dress it all with my homemade ranch, which we always have on hand to use throughout the week. This dish is simple, nourishing, and flavorful.

---

4 medium Yukon Gold potatoes

FOR ROASTING/AIR-FRYING (OPTIONAL)
¼ cup fresh lemon juice (from about 1 lemon)
2 teaspoons dried oregano
1 teaspoon sea salt, plus more as needed
1 teaspoon onion powder
1 teaspoon garlic powder
½ teaspoon dried thyme

TO SERVE
8 cups arugula or spring greens
1 cup canned white beans, such as cannellini or navy, drained and rinsed
¼ cup thinly sliced red onion
½ cup Cashew Ranch Dressing (page 181)

---

1. Place the potatoes in a small pot and add enough cold water to just cover them. Bring the water to a boil over high heat, then reduce the heat to maintain a simmer. Cook the potatoes until they can be easily pierced with a fork, 15 to 20 minutes. (Alternatively, steam the potatoes on the stovetop or in the microwave for 10 to 15 minutes.)

2. **For the roasted or air-fried version:** Preheat the oven or air fryer to 425°F. If roasting, line a baking sheet with parchment paper.

3. In a large bowl, combine the potatoes, lemon juice, oregano, salt, onion powder, garlic powder, and thyme. Toss until the potatoes are evenly coated. Spread the potatoes in a single layer over the prepared baking sheet or in the basket of the air fryer. Roast for 15 minutes or air-fry for 10 minutes, until the potatoes are crispy.

4. Create a bed of the greens on a plate or in a bowl. Top with the potatoes, beans, and onion. Toss with the ranch dressing and serve.

> **NOTE:** I've shared two ways to make this recipe: a quick way, and a roasted/air-fried way. Both offer an easy, nourishing meal with great flavor, but the roasted version kicks it up a notch—go with whichever works best for you!

NUTRITION INFORMATION
SERVING SIZE: 1 serving   **CALORIES:** 532   **PROTEIN:** 20 g   **CARBS:** 87 g   **FAT:** 7 g

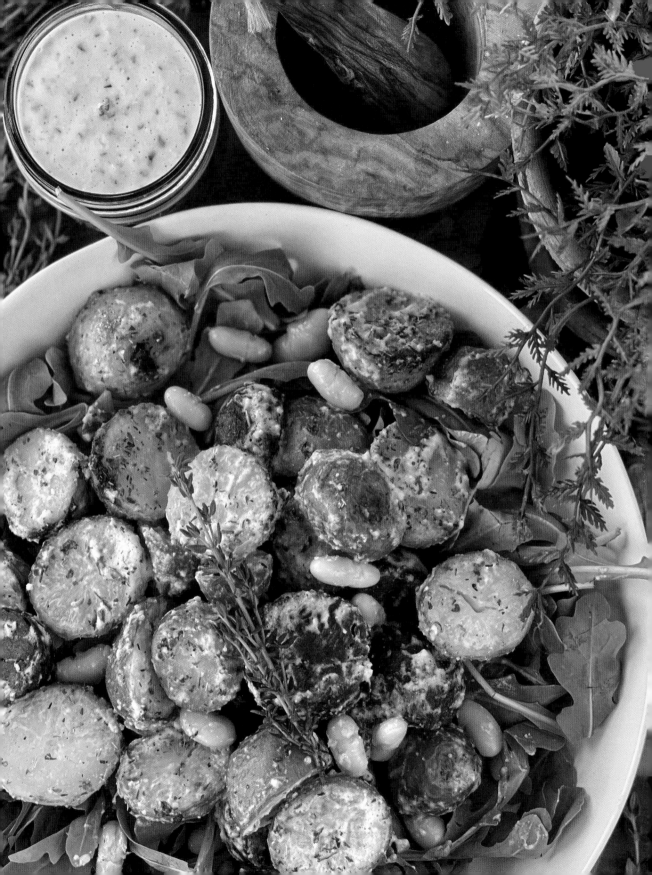

Garlic Rosemary Roasted Sweet Potatoes with Raspberry-Lime Sauce

SERVES 2

There's something magical about the combination of sweet potato and raspberry jelly. The rosemary adds a savory note to this simple dish and pairs well with a salad or a side of steamed asparagus. You can cook your potatoes ahead when you're batch prepping for the week and shave off a lot of time from this recipe.

---

2 large sweet potatoes (see Note)
Fresh lemon juice
2 tablespoons nutritional yeast (optional; see Note)
½ teaspoon garlic powder
**½ teaspoon garlic salt, plus more
if you like things garlicky**
¼ teaspoon ground rosemary
2 tablespoons Raspberry-Lime Sauce (page 191)

---

1. Preheat the oven to 425°F. Line a baking sheet with parchment paper.

2. Slice the sweet potatoes into the fry shape of your choice (I like to cut mine into ½-inch-thick spears). Spread the fries over the prepared baking sheet and squeeze lemon juice over them. Season with the nutritional yeast (if using), garlic powder, garlic salt, and rosemary. Toss to evenly coat the potatoes.

3. Bake for 30 to 40 minutes, until crisp. Serve with the raspberry-lime sauce.

NOTE: If you roast or steam your potatoes in advance, reduce the cooking time to 20 to 30 minutes. Nutritional yeast (not to be confused with brewer's yeast) is a type of deactivated yeast. It has a nutty, cheesy flavor and is often used in place of cheese in plant-based cooking. It's also a significant source of B vitamins.

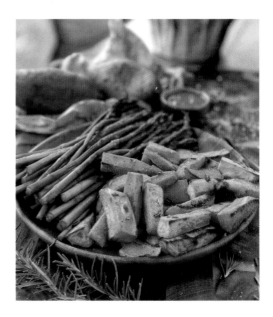

NUTRITION INFORMATION
SERVING SIZE: 1 serving **CALORIES:** 440 **PROTEIN:** 13 g **CARBS:** 83 g **FAT:** 1 g

Philly "Cheesesteak" Spuds

My husband thought for sure he would never be able to give up meat, so I started making this cheesesteak sandwich filled with mushroom "meat" that he absolutely loves. But one day, I didn't have any bread in the house and we don't live in town, so I improvised and used baked potatoes instead of bread, and the mushroom filling went on top of the potatoes. It was another hit!

---

4 medium Yukon Gold potatoes
16 ounces portobello mushrooms, sliced
2 green bell peppers, sliced
1 medium yellow onion, sliced
1 teaspoon garlic powder or minced fresh garlic
Pinch of sea salt
2 tablespoons vegan Worcestershire sauce (I like Annie's)
1 cup Cheese Sauce (page 176), warmed

---

1. Place the potatoes in a small pot and add enough cold water to just cover them. Bring the water to a boil over medium-high heat, then reduce the heat to maintain a simmer. Cook the potatoes until they can be easily pierced with a fork, 15 to 20 minutes. (Alternatively, steam the potatoes on the stovetop or in the microwave for 10 to 15 minutes, or roast them in a 425°F oven for 40 minutes.)

2. In a large nonstick sauté pan, combine the mushrooms, peppers, and onion. Season with the garlic powder and salt and cook over medium-high heat, stirring only very occasionally, until softened, 8 to 10 minutes. If needed, add a few tablespoons of water to the pan to help the vegetables cook down. Stir in the Worcestershire and remove the pan from the heat.

3. When the potatoes are cool enough to handle, slice them in half and use a fork to smash them slightly. Top the potatoes with the vegetable mixture and the cheese sauce and serve.

NUTRITION INFORMATION
SERVING SIZE: 1 serving   **CALORIES:** 494   **PROTEIN:** 13 g   **CARBS:** 90 g   **FAT:** 5 g

Lemon Greek Potatoes

SERVES
2

There was a little Greek café in downtown Boulder whose fries I loved. The restaurant was just a little hole-in-the-wall run by the owner and his wife, and the place always smelled delicious. My favorite thing on the menu was their fries. They were well seasoned with garlic and oregano, and sprinkled with lemon juice just before serving. The café had a bright and creamy herbed yogurt dip that they served on the side. I was always going back for more. This is my take on those Greek fries, and they're so good that I don't miss the ones that inspired this recipe. Don't be afraid to spray these with a little oil to help them crisp up, especially if you're new to oil-free vegan cooking. A light spray of oil goes a long way, and it won't sabotage your weight loss.

4 medium Yukon Gold potatoes
¼ cup fresh lemon juice (from about 1 lemon)
1 teaspoon dried oregano
½ teaspoon onion powder
½ teaspoon garlic powder
½ teaspoon sea salt
Pinch of ground turmeric (optional, for color)
¼ cup Cashew Ranch Dressing (page 181) or ketchup, for serving

1. Preheat the oven or air fryer to 425°F. If roasting in the oven, line a baking sheet with parchment paper.

2. Place the potatoes in a small pot and add enough cold water just to cover them. Bring the water to a boil over medium-high heat, then reduce the heat to maintain a simmer. Cook the potatoes until they can be easily pierced with a fork, 15 to 20 minutes. (Alternatively, steam the potatoes on the stovetop or in the microwave for 10 to 15 minutes.)

3. Transfer the potatoes to a food storage container with a lid. Top with the lemon juice, oregano, onion powder, garlic powder, salt, and turmeric (if using). Close the container and give the potatoes a vigorous shake so that they're well coated and a bit roughed up, which will help them get crisp in the oven.

4. Spread the potatoes in a single layer over the prepared baking sheet or in the basket of your air fryer and cook until the potatoes are golden and crisp, 15 to 20 minutes in the oven or 10 to 15 minutes in the air fryer.

5. Enjoy with ranch dressing or ketchup.

NUTRITION INFORMATION
SERVING SIZE: 1 serving (not including ranch dressing; see page 181 for nutrition information)   **CALORIES:** 315
PROTEIN: 7 g   **CARBS:** 65 g   **FAT:** 0.5 g

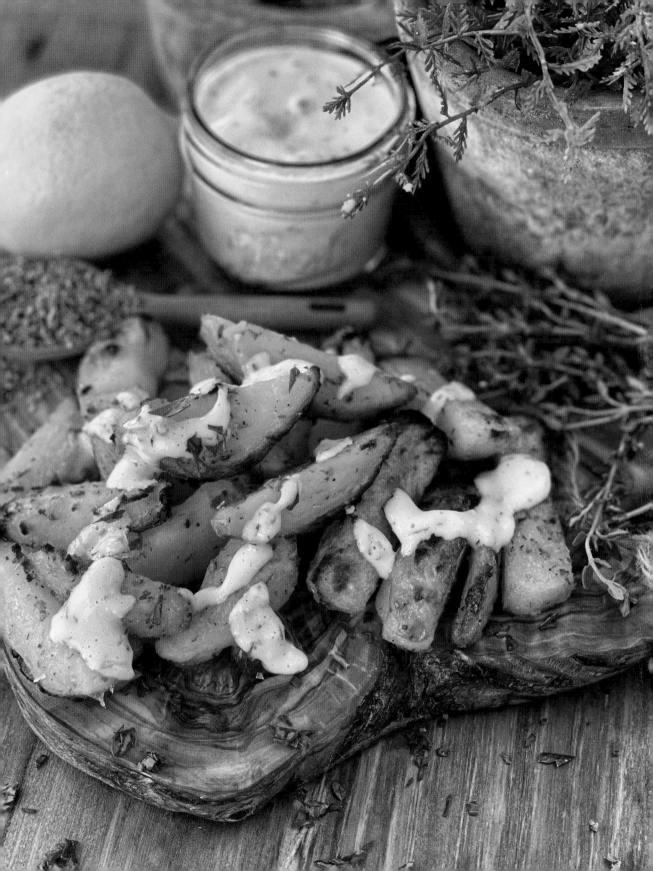

Curry Hummus Sammy

I love veggie-filled sandwiches with delicious spreads. This curry hummus adds so much flavor and depth to an otherwise simple sandwich. You can try adding a few thin slices of avocado for an even richer and creamier flavor. Any leftover hummus can be used as a dip for veggies for a nutritious snack.

NOTE: My favorite bread is Ezekiel 4:9 sprouted whole-grain bread; for a gluten-free option, I'll use Outside the Breadbox vegan oat bread. Feel free to use what you like.

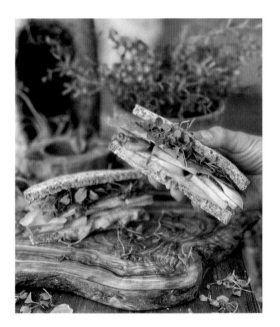

4 slices sprouted whole-grain bread or gluten-free bread (see Note), toasted

½ cup Cilantro-Curry Hummus (page 195)

1 medium English cucumber, sliced

2 Roma (plum) tomatoes, sliced

8 romaine lettuce leaves

1 cup microgreens or sprouts

1. Place two slices of the toast on a clean work surface.

2. Spread half the hummus over each slice, then layer on the cucumber, tomatoes, lettuce, and microgreens, dividing them evenly. Top each with a second slice of toast and serve.

NUTRITION INFORMATION
SERVING SIZE: 1 sandwich   **CALORIES:** 264   **PROTEIN:** 15 g   **CARBS:** 34 g   **FAT:** 1 g

Buffalo Chickpea Salad Wrap

MAKES
2
WRAPS

Wraps at lunchtime always sound good to me. I like mine fully loaded with fresh vegetables and dressed with a savory, creamy dressing. If you keep sliced cucumbers and fresh greens in the fridge, cleaned and ready to grab, you can throw together this wrap in a matter of minutes. If you'd like to forgo the wrap, try serving all the fillings on a bed of greens for a tasty and filling salad.

NOTE: When it comes to finding oil-free flour tortillas, I've never had much luck. That's why I go with the next best thing: a tortilla that's low in fat and calories (Olé Mexican Foods Xtreme Wellness wraps are my favorite). You can also look for oil-free lavash wraps, which are a little harder to come by but a delicious option. Or you could change the recipe slightly and either substitute your favorite bread to turn this into a sandwich, or heap everything on top of the greens in a bowl.

2 (10-inch) flour tortillas or gluten-free wraps (see Note)

1 cup Buffalo Chickpea Dip (page 209)

2 cups spring greens, or 2 romaine lettuce leaves

1 medium English cucumber, sliced

2 Roma (plum) tomatoes, sliced

¼ cup thinly sliced red onion

½ small avocado, sliced (optional)

¼ cup Cashew Ranch Dressing (page 181)

1. Place the tortillas on a clean work surface.

2. Dollop the Buffalo chickpea dip down the middle of each wrap. Layer the greens, cucumber, tomatoes, onion, and avocado (if using) on top.

3. Drizzle with the ranch dressing and roll up the tortillas to enclose the filling.

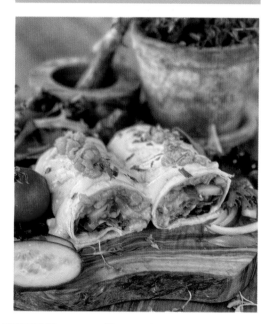

NUTRITION INFORMATION
SERVING SIZE: 1 wrap (not including avocado)   **CALORIES:** 330   **PROTEIN:** 18 g   **CARBS:** 35 g   **FAT:** 9 g

IF ADDING ¼ SMALL AVOCADO, ADD:
CALORIES: 43   **PROTEIN:** 0.5 g   **CARBS:** 0.5 g   **FAT:** 4 g

Eggless Egg Salad Sammy

My mom used to make me egg salad sandwiches all the time, and they were my favorite packed-lunch option for school. I decided to try making my own plant-based version with chickpeas, and the result was this fiber-filled, cholesterol-free, and easy-to-pack "egg" salad. Best of all, I can bring it on a hot-day hike without worrying about it spoiling quickly the way the traditional kind would.

> **NOTE:** My favorite bread is Ezekiel 4:9 sprouted whole-grain bread; for a gluten-free option, I'll use Outside the Breadbox vegan oat bread, but feel free to use what you like.

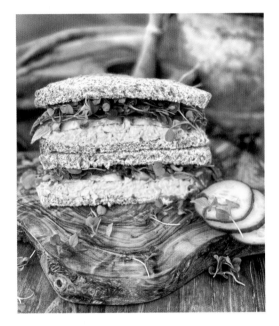

4 slices sprouted whole-grain bread or gluten-free bread (see Note), toasted

1 cup Easy Eggless Egg Salad (page 200)

8 romaine lettuce leaves

1 small English cucumber, sliced

1 cup microgreens or sprouts

½ small avocado, sliced (optional)

1. Place 2 slices of the toast on a clean work surface and spread them with the egg salad, dividing it evenly.

2. Top each with half the lettuce, cucumber, microgreens, and avocado (if using). Close each sandwich with a second slice of toast and enjoy.

NUTRITION INFORMATION
SERVING SIZE: 1 sandwich (not including avocado) **CALORIES:** 380 **PROTEIN:** 19 g **CARBS:** 47 g **FAT:** 7 g

IF ADDING ¼ SMALL AVOCADO, ADD:
CALORIES: 43 **PROTEIN:** 0.5 g **CARBS:** 0.5 g **FAT:** 4 g

Chickpea "Chicken" Salad Sammy

This sandwich is a favorite in our house, and it's the one we pack for picnics, hikes, and road trips! Everyone loves the creamy flavor and the crunch from adding some diced celery and red onion to the "chicken" salad. This makes a great cold lunch option for those of you who don't have a way to heat up your lunch at work or need something to grab quickly and take on the go.

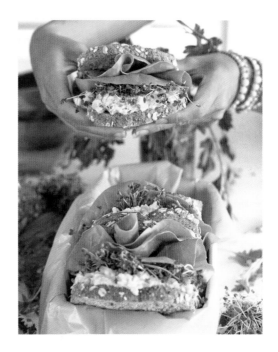

4 slices sprouted whole-grain bread or gluten-free bread (see Note opposite), toasted

1 cup Chickpea "Chicken" Salad (page 203)

8 romaine lettuce leaves

1 cup sprouts or microgreens

1. Place 2 slices of the toast on a clean work surface and spread them with the chicken salad, dividing it evenly.

2. Top with the lettuce and sprouts, add a second slice of toast to each, and serve.

NUTRITION INFORMATION
SERVING SIZE: 1 sandwich   **CALORIES:** 411   **PROTEIN:** 20 g   **CARBS:** 53 g   **FAT:** 10 g

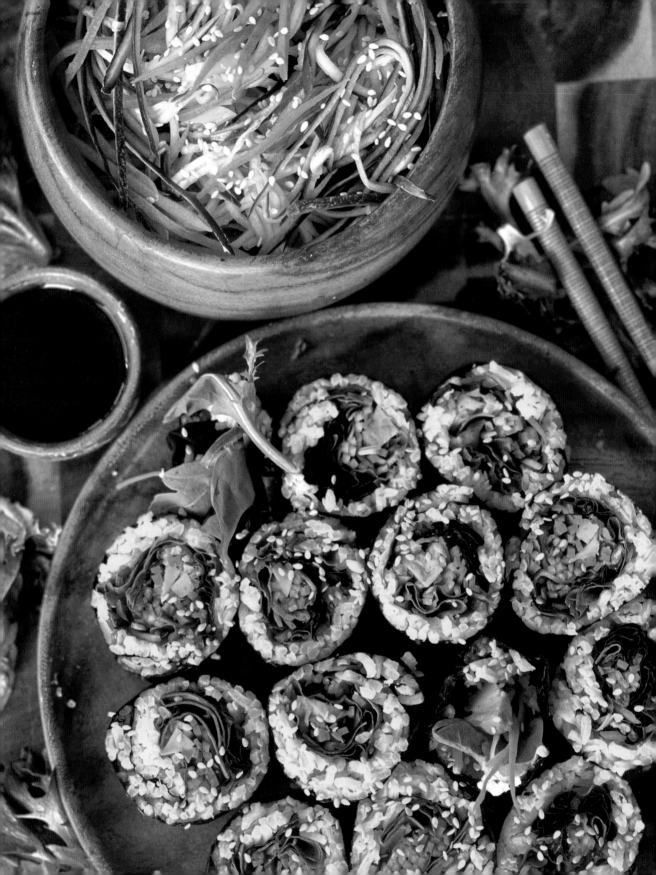

Sushi

MAKES
4
ROLLS

Sushi is my obsession—every week when it's date night and my husband asks what I'm in the mood to eat, my answer is almost always sushi. This sushi is surprisingly easy to make at home and requires no special folding mats or other tools. To make my rice sticky so it rolls up well in the nori sheets without falling out, I just add an extra ¼ to ½ cup of water while it cooks. Try adding mango or sweet potato to your rolls—both will give them even more flavor, which will give you more satisfaction.

---

3 cups jasmine rice

4 nori sheets

2 cups spring greens

1 large English cucumber, cut into thin matchsticks

2 large carrots, cut into thin matchsticks

1 small avocado, sliced (optional)

1 medium mango or cooked sweet potato, sliced into thin matchsticks (optional)

Sesame seeds, for garnish (optional)

Low-sodium soy sauce or coconut aminos, for serving

---

1. Cook the rice according to the package instructions, using an additional ½ cup water (this will help make the rice sticky). Remove from the heat and let the rice cool completely; hot rice will make your nori soggy and cause it tear.

2. Place 1 nori sheet on a cutting board. Add ¾ cup of the rice and use your hands to gently press it into a smooth, even layer, leaving a ½-inch border at the top of the sheet. If you skip this step, it will be difficult to seal your sushi roll. At the bottom edge of the roll, layer one-quarter of the greens, cucumber, carrots, and, if desired, avocado and mango over the rice.

3. Using a wet fingertip, lightly dampen the exposed edges of the nori. Starting from the bottom, begin rolling up the nori around the fillings. The trick is to get it nice and tight without tearing the nori. (Don't worry, even the messy-looking rolls taste delicious!) Use a sharp knife to slice the roll crosswise into bite-size pieces and set aside on a plate. Repeat with the remaining ingredients to make 3 additional rolls.

4. Garnish the rolls with sesame seeds, if desired, and serve with soy sauce or coconut aminos for dipping.

NUTRITION INFORMATION
SERVING SIZE: 2 rolls (with avocado)   **CALORIES:** 408   **PROTEIN:** 11 g   **CARBS:** 70 g   **FAT:** 6 g

Smoky Tomato Hummus Wrap

MAKES
2
WRAPS

This is another favorite wrap. The smoky BBQ Ranch takes it to the next level, but you could use whatever dressing you decided to prep for the week and it'll still be delicious! I like having this with a salad or a bowl of fresh fruit.

2 small Yukon Gold potatoes

2 (10-inch) spinach tortillas, flour tortillas, or gluten-free wraps (see Note)

½ cup Smoky Tomato Hummus (page 196)

2 cups spring greens

1 Roma (plum) tomato, sliced

¼ cup thinly sliced red onion

½ small avocado, sliced (optional)

¼ cup BBQ Ranch (page 178)

2 tablespoons chopped fresh cilantro leaves

1. Place the potatoes in a small microwave-safe dish with a fitted lid, add 1 teaspoon water, and cover. Microwave for 6 to 8 minutes, until the potatoes are tender. Slice the potatoes into wedges or use the bottom of a glass or the flat side of a large knife to smash them.

2. Lay the tortillas on a clean work surface. Dollop the hummus down the center of each tortilla and top evenly with the steamed potato, greens, tomato, onion, and avocado, if desired. Drizzle with the ranch and sprinkle with the cilantro. Roll up the wraps to enclose the filling and serve.

NOTE: For a low-calorie wrap option, I like Olé Mexican Foods Xtreme Wellness wraps.

NUTRITION INFORMATION
SERVING SIZE: 1 wrap (not including avocado)   **CALORIES:** 336   **PROTEIN:** 16 g   **CARBS:** 47 g   **FAT:** 6 g

IF ADDING ¼ SMALL AVOCADO, ADD:
CALORIES: 43   **PROTEIN:** 0.5 g   **CARBS:** 0.5 g   **FAT:** 4 g

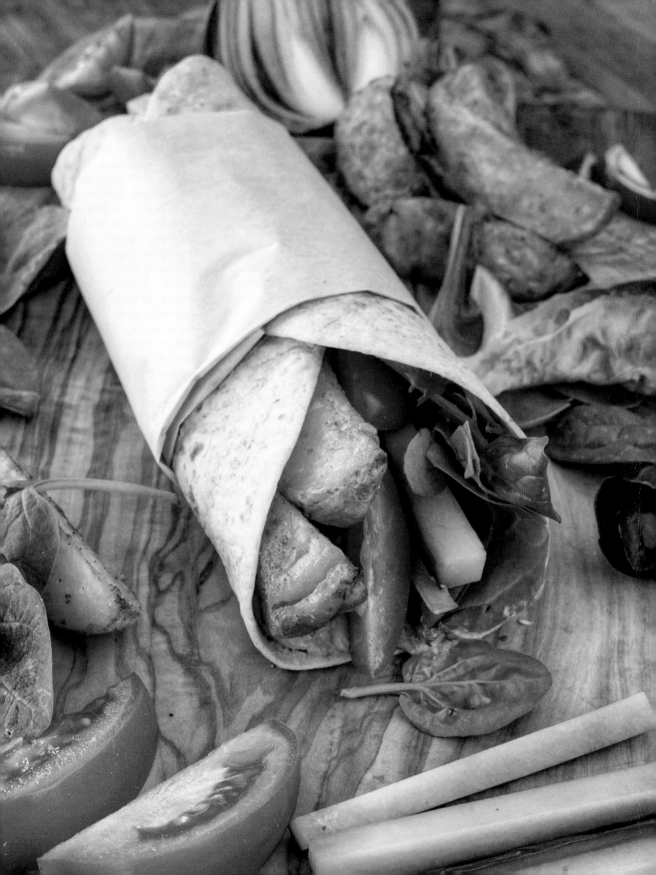

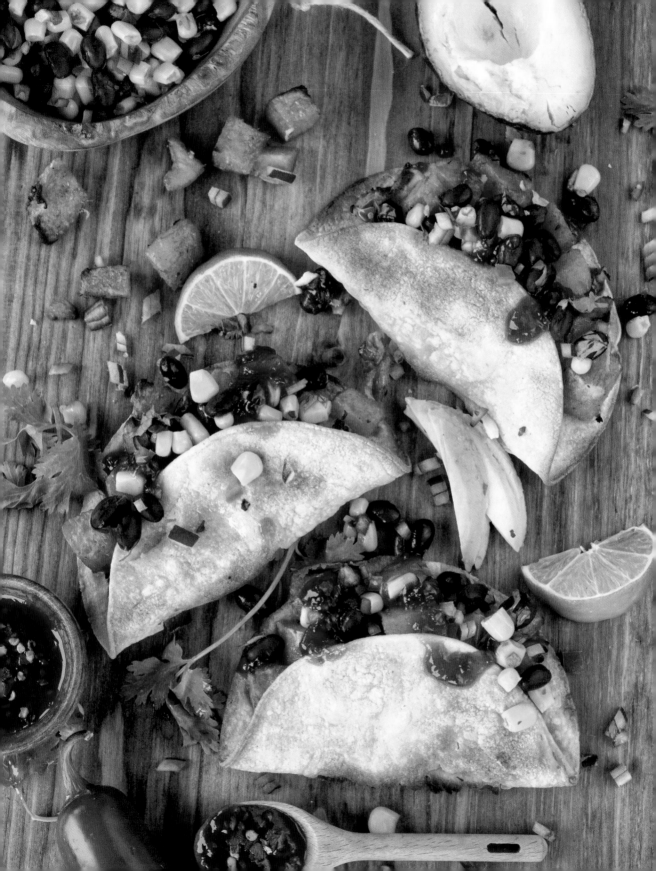

Sweet Potato Tacos

MAKES
6
TACOS

So, I have a confession: Sweet potatoes are probably my least favorite food, closely followed by cauliflower. But I've always known how good they are for my health, so I kept trying to like them. These tacos are the first way I enjoyed eating sweet potatoes. The combination of chili, onion, and paprika with a hint of sweet raspberry and lime is incredible. This is another meal that can be prepped ahead of time and then assembled and heated when you're ready to eat.

1. Preheat the oven to 425°F. Line a baking sheet with parchment paper.

2. Spread the sweet potato cubes over the prepared baking sheet. Sprinkle the lime juice over the potatoes and season with the paprika, garlic salt, chili powder, and onion powder. Toss to coat the potatoes well. Roast for 30 to 40 minutes, until the potatoes are tender and beginning to brown.

3. To serve, bundle the spiced sweet potatoes into the tortillas and top with the salsa, raspberry-lime sauce, and avocado, if desired.

2 large sweet potatoes, cut into 1-inch cubes

Juice of ½ lime

½ teaspoon smoked paprika

½ teaspoon garlic salt, or to taste

¼ teaspoon chili powder

¼ teaspoon onion powder

6 (8-inch) corn tortillas, warmed, or 6 romaine lettuce leaves (see Note)

1 cup Black Bean Salsa (page 213)

¼ cup Raspberry-Lime Sauce (page 191)

½ small avocado, sliced (optional)

NOTE: To reduce the calorie density of these tacos, turn them into lettuce boats instead—just swap the corn tortillas for romaine lettuce leaves.

NUTRITION INFORMATION

SERVING SIZE: 3 tacos on corn tortillas (not including avocado)   CALORIES: 595   PROTEIN: 45 g   CARBS: 113 g   FAT: 3 g

SERVING SIZE: 3 tacos on lettuce leaves (not including avocado)   CALORIES: 430   PROTEIN: 10 g   CARBS: 89 g   FAT: 1 g

IF ADDING ¼ SMALL AVOCADO, ADD:

CALORIES: 43   PROTEIN: 0.5 g   CARBS: 0.5 g   FAT: 4 g

Masa Cakes

I'm half Mayan and was born in the Yucatán, so it's no surprise that I'm drawn to traditional Mayan food, which is full of flavor and always involves masa harina, beans, and pickled onions. Don't leave out the pickled onions—they add such amazing flavor to this dish, as well as to burrito bowls and even avocado toast!

---

1 cup masa harina
All-purpose flour (optional)
Avocado oil cooking spray (optional)
1 cup fat-free refried beans, store bought or homemade
½ cup salsa, store-bought or homemade
½ cup Pickled Onions (page 188)
½ small avocado, sliced (optional)
Fresh lime juice

---

1. In a small bowl, mix the masa with ½ cup water until it comes together to make a dough. The dough should hold together without being too wet or crumbly; you may need to add more water a tablespoon at a time to get the dough to come together.

2. Form the dough into 3 equal-size balls. Sandwich one ball at a time between two sheets of parchment paper and use the palm of your hand to gently flatten the ball until it's roughly ½ inch thick. They should look like thick tortillas. Reuse the parchment paper to flatten the remaining two balls. (Alternatively, dust a clean work surface and the dough balls with flour and use a rolling pin to flatten them.)

3. Heat a nonstick griddle or skillet over medium heat. Lightly coat the pan with cooking spray, if yours likes to stick. Carefully remove the masa cakes from the parchment and place them on the griddle. Cook for about 3 minutes, until the bottoms begin to brown. Flip and cook for about 3 minutes more, until the second side has begun to brown. Transfer the cooked masa cakes to a plate.

4. Top the cakes with the refried beans, salsa, pickled onions, and avocado, if desired. Squeeze some lime juice over the top and serve.

NUTRITION INFORMATION
SERVING SIZE: 1 serving (including avocado)   **CALORIES:** 395   **PROTEIN:** 14 g   **CARBS:** 57 g   **FAT:** 8 g

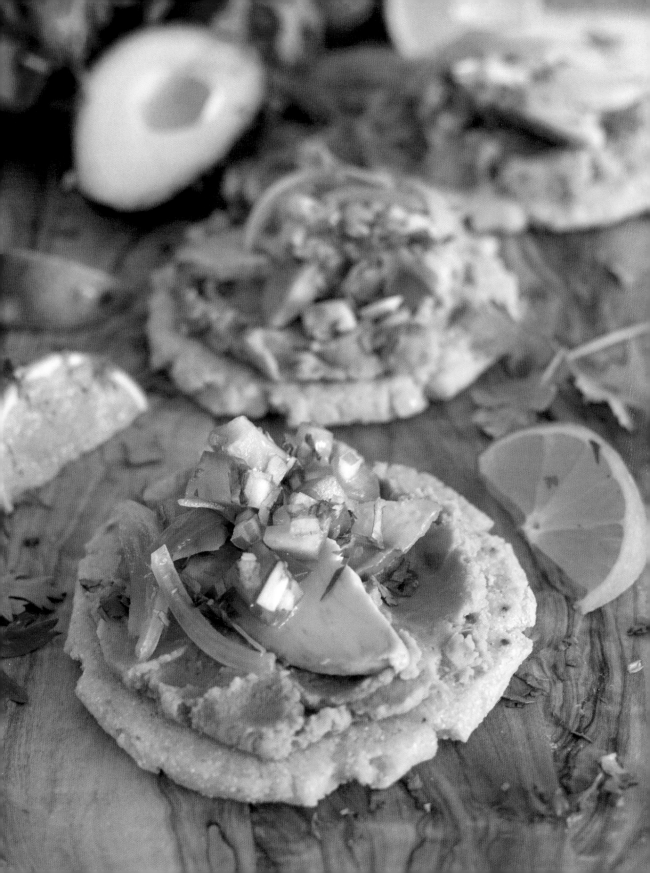

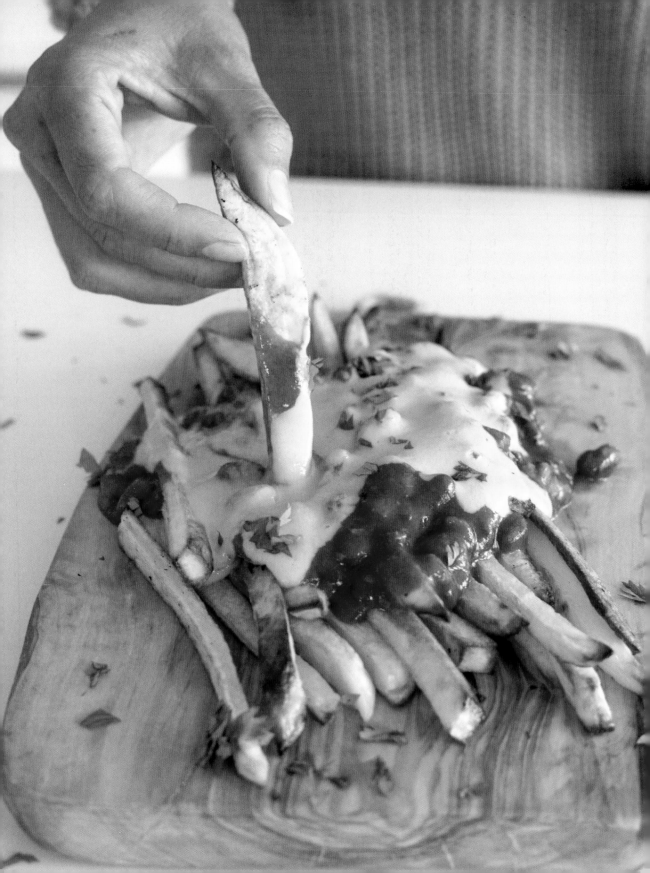

Chili Cheese Fries

SERVES

2

Even though half my roots are in the Yucatán, my mother is American, and I grew up in beautiful Colorado. During the summer, it was a family tradition to visit the county fair, and I always looked forward to a paper plate full of chili cheese fries. (Great for their taste, but not so much for one's health.) I've cleaned up this old-school favorite, and—I promise you—it still tastes just like the county fair fries I loved so much as a kid. Using canned vegetable chili makes this dish super easy, but if you have homemade chili on hand, feel free to sub that in! If you do use store-bought chili, just look for one that's fat-free or as low in fat as possible, with around 200 calories or fewer per cup.

4 medium Yukon Gold potatoes (see Note)

½ teaspoon garlic salt, or to taste

1 cup canned low-fat or fat-free vegetable chili (I like Hormel vegetarian chili with beans), warmed

½ cup Cheese Sauce (page 176), warmed

1. Preheat the oven to 425°F. Line a baking sheet with parchment paper.

2. Slice the potatoes into your desired fry shape (I like to cut mine into ½-inch-thick spears). Spread the fries in a single layer on the prepared baking sheet and sprinkle with the garlic salt. Toss to coat well. Roast for 20 to 30 minutes, until crispy.

3. Top with the warmed chili and cheese sauce and serve.

> **NOTE:** You can make these fries from raw potatoes, or use leftover cooked potatoes.

NUTRITION INFORMATION
SERVING SIZE: 1 serving **CALORIES:** 458 **PROTEIN:** 13 g **CARBS:** 83 g **FAT:** 3 g

Cheesy Broccoli Rice Casserole

If you grew up in the '80s and early '90s, chances are, you ate your fair share of casseroles like I did. And what's not to love about a casserole? They're easy to put together and generally crowd pleasers. This one is no different—my family loves it! If you have the cheese sauce prepped ahead of time and some rice already steamed, all you have to do is add some steamed or roasted broccoli to the rice, mix in the sauce, and you're ready to go. The bread crumb topping adds a delicious, satisfying crunch.

4 cups broccoli florets
4 cups white or brown rice, cooked
1 cup Cheese Sauce (page 176), warmed
½ teaspoon garlic salt, plus more as needed
Freshly ground black pepper
¼ cup Panko bread crumbs

1. If you'll be including the bread crumb topping, preheat the oven to 425°F.

2. Fill a medium pot with a fitted lid with 2 inches of water and bring to a simmer over medium-high heat. Put the broccoli in a steamer basket and place it in the pot. Cover the pot and steam for 6 minutes, until the broccoli is bright green and tender but not mushy. (Alternatively, put the broccoli in a microwave-safe container, add 1 tablespoon water, cover, and microwave for 4 minutes.)

3. Finely chop the broccoli and transfer it to a medium bowl. Add the cooked rice, cheese sauce, and garlic salt, season with pepper, and enjoy. If using bread crumbs, combine the chopped broccoli, cooked rice, cheese sauce, and garlic salt in an oven-safe dish and season with pepper. Sprinkle evenly with the bread crumbs and a pinch more garlic salt and bake for 15 to 20 minutes, until the bread crumbs are toasted, then serve.

NUTRITION INFORMATION
SERVING SIZE: 1 serving (not including the bread crumbs)   **CALORIES:** 578   **PROTEIN:** 18 g   **CARBS:** 109 g   **FAT:** 4 g

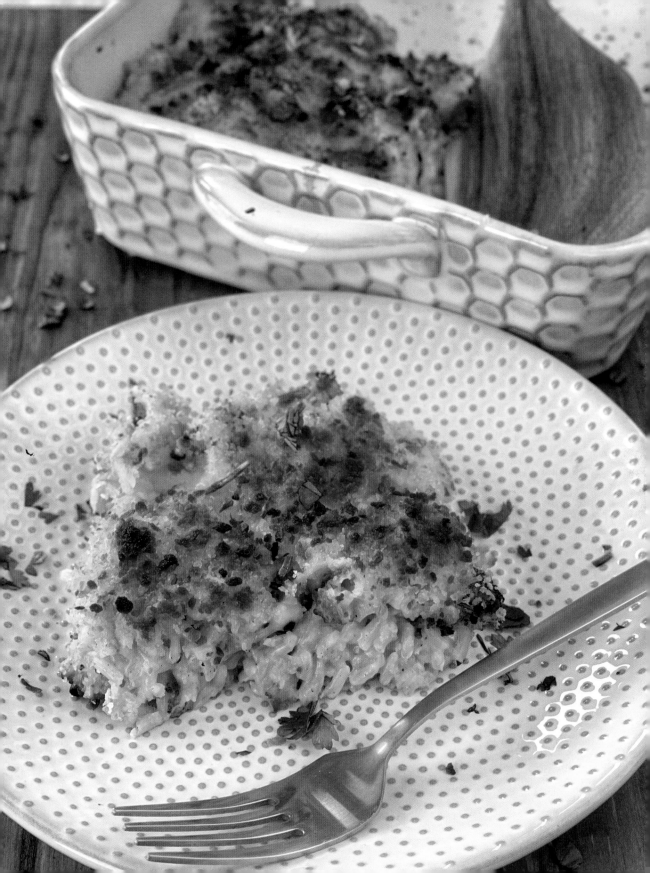

Smoky Maple-Roasted Sweet Potato Fries

Colorado mountain towns are known not only for their amazing trails and skiing but also for their breweries and pub food. Sweet potato fries can be found at almost every pub I've ever visited, and they never disappoint. I decided to make my own non-fried version; the smoked paprika and maple syrup put them over the top! Garlic salt is preferable here since it won't melt into the fries, but if you don't have it on hand, seasoning with garlic powder is a good substitute. And cooking the potatoes ahead during meal prep makes this recipe even easier.

---

2 large sweet potatoes (see Note)

Fresh lemon juice

½ teaspoon smoked paprika

½ teaspoon garlic salt, or more, if you like things garlicky

2 tablespoons pure maple syrup

---

1. Preheat the oven to 425°F. Line a baking sheet with parchment paper.

2. Slice the sweet potatoes into the fry shape of your choice (I like cutting mine into ¼-inch-thick spears). Spread the fries over the prepared baking sheet and squeeze lemon juice over them. Season with the paprika and garlic salt. Toss to evenly coat the potatoes.

3. Bake for 30 to 40 minutes, until the fries are beginning to brown. Remove from the oven, drizzle with the maple syrup, and toss to coat. Serve warm.

> **NOTE:** If you roast or steam your potatoes in advance, reduce the cooking time to 20 to 30 minutes.

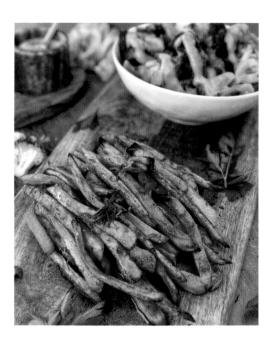

NUTRITION INFORMATION

SERVING SIZE: 1 serving   **CALORIES:** 413   **PROTEIN:** 8 g   **CARBS:** 83 g   **FAT:** 1 g

Loaded Baked Potatoes

Remember when soup-and-salad buffets were everywhere? I would always get loaded baked potatoes and some salad. So satisfying. These potatoes make an easy, comforting weeknight dinner, and if you make your cheese sauce ahead of time and precook your potatoes, you're just assembling and adding any toppings that you've already prepped or saved from leftovers.

4 medium russet potatoes

4 cups broccoli florets

8 ounces baby bella (cremini) mushrooms, sliced or quartered

Sea salt and freshly ground black pepper

1 cup Cheese Sauce (page 176), warmed

2 green onions, white and green parts sliced

Ketchup, for serving (optional)

Parsley, for garnish (optional)

1. Preheat the oven to 425°F. Line a baking sheet with parchment paper.

2. Set the potato on the prepared baking sheet. Bake for 45 minutes, or until a knife can easily be inserted into the center. (Alternatively, cook the potato in a pressure cooker on high pressure for 20 minutes.)

3. Meanwhile, fill a medium pot with a fitted lid with 2 inches of water and bring to a simmer over medium-high heat. Put the broccoli in a steamer basket and place it in the pot. Cover the pot and steam for 6 minutes, until the broccoli is bright green and tender but not mushy. (Alternatively, put the broccoli in a microwave-safe container, add 1 tablespoon water, cover, and microwave for 4 minutes.)

4. In a large nonstick sauté pan, cook the mushrooms over medium heat. Add a splash of water to help them soften, if necessary. Continue cooking until the mushrooms are beginning to brown, about 8 minutes. Taste and season with salt and pepper.

5. To serve, slice or mash the potatoes, then top them with the steamed broccoli, sautéed mushrooms, cheese sauce, green onions, and, if you want to try it our way, a drizzle of ketchup.

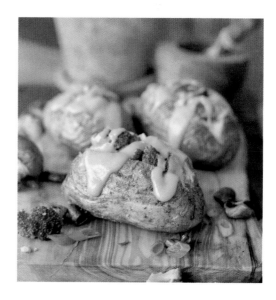

NUTRITION INFORMATION

SERVING SIZE: 1 serving **CALORIES:** 553 **PROTEIN:** 20 g **CARBS:** 96 g **FAT:** 4 g

Shiitake Rice with Bok Choy and Thai Peanut Sauce

SERVES
2

Sometimes simple meals are the most delicious meals, and this is one of those—even my kids love it. I give them teriyaki seaweed to eat with it, which takes this to a whole new level, adding a sweet, tangy, and salty crunch to the dish. If you don't have time to make the peanut dressing or if it's just not your thing, just add some coconut aminos teriyaki sauce on top, and it'll be every bit as delicious!

2 pounds baby bok choy, ends trimmed

8 ounces shiitake mushrooms, sliced

4 cups white or brown rice, cooked

¼ cup Thai Peanut Sauce (page 183)
or coconut aminos teriyaki sauce
(I like Coconut Secret)

2 green onions, white and green parts sliced

2 tablespoons chopped fresh cilantro leaves

1. In a large nonstick pan, combine the bok choy and mushrooms. Cook over medium heat until softened and tender, adding a splash of water to the pan if necessary, about 3 minutes.

2. Divide the rice between two bowls and top with the sautéed veggies, peanut sauce or coconut aminos, green onions, and cilantro, then serve.

NUTRITION INFORMATION
SERVING SIZE: 1 serving   **CALORIES:** 582   **PROTEIN:** 24 g   **CARBS:** 106 g   **FAT:** 4 g

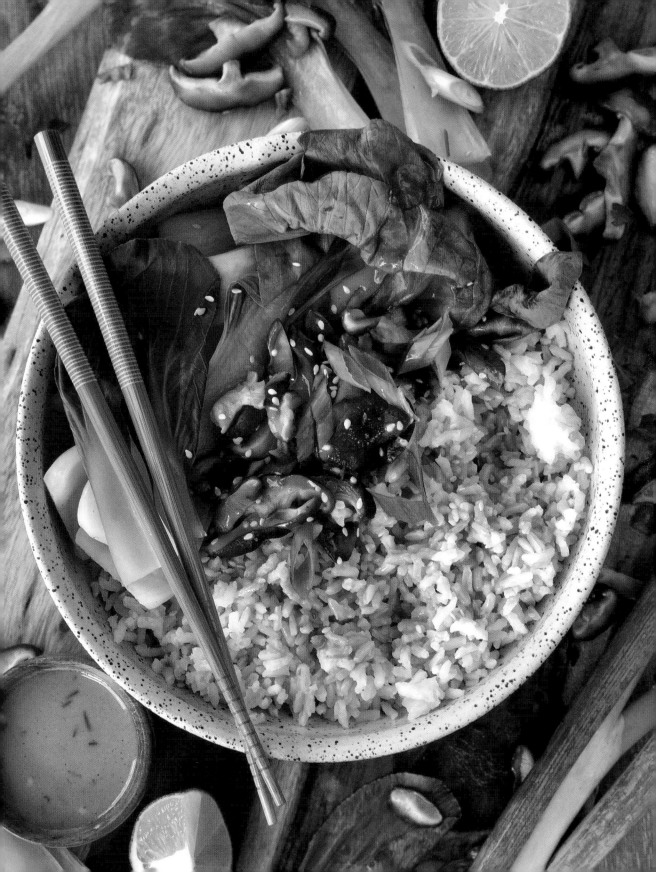

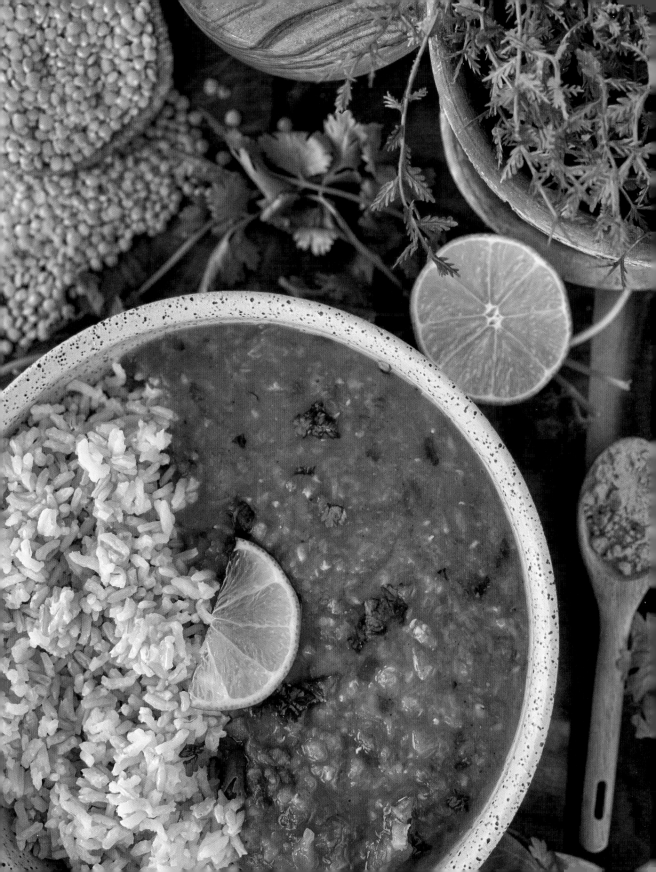

Easy Lentil Curry

SERVES
4

This is one of my favorite dishes for two reasons. First, it's a curry, and second, my Instant Pot does all the work. This is meant to be more like a soup that goes over steamed rice than a thick stew. Adding a little lime and cilantro at the end brightens the dish and bumps up the flavor. Best of all, the curry can stay in the fridge all week for leftovers and it's great for freezing.

⅛ teaspoon cumin seeds
2 Roma (plum) tomatoes, diced
1 medium yellow onion, diced
1 tablespoon minced garlic
2 teaspoons garam masala
1 teaspoon curry powder
1 teaspoon ground coriander
1 teaspoon sea salt
½ teaspoon minced fresh ginger
1 cup dried red lentils
4 cups white or brown rice, cooked, for serving
Chopped fresh cilantro leaves, for garnish
Fresh lime juice

1. Select the Sauté setting on your Instant Pot or multicooker. Place the cumin seeds in the inner pot and toast until fragrant and browned, about 1 minute. Add the tomatoes, onion, garlic, garam masala, curry powder, coriander, salt, and ginger. Cook, stirring occasionally, for 5 minutes.

2. Stir in the lentils plus 5 cups water. Seal the pot and pressure-cook for 20 minutes, then allow the pressure to release naturally.

3. Serve the lentils over the rice, topped with cilantro and a squeeze of lime juice. Store any leftovers in an airtight container in the refrigerator for up to a week, or freeze for up to a month. The curry is even more delicious the next day!

NUTRITION INFORMATION
SERVING SIZE: 1½ cups curry with 1 cup steamed rice   **CALORIES:** 544   **PROTEIN:** 28 g   **CARBS:** 92 g   **FAT:** 3 g

⑤⅝ Spring Roll Bowl

This bowl is perfect for anyone who loves the crunch and lightness of fresh spring rolls (especially if they love the salty umami of soy sauce) but is not great at wrapping them. I like to prepare all the ingredients for this salad ahead of time and keep them in containers in my fridge so I can throw a bowl together with ease a few times during the week.

¼ cup coconut aminos teriyaki sauce (I like Coconut Secret) or 2 tablespoons seasoned rice vinegar plus 2 tablespoons low-sodium soy sauce

2 cups white or brown rice, cooked

8 cups spring greens

2 medium carrots, sliced into thin matchsticks

1 medium English cucumber, sliced into thin matchsticks

1 cup sliced fresh mango

½ small avocado, sliced (optional)

2 green onions, white and green parts sliced

¼ cup thinly sliced red onion

¼ cup chopped fresh cilantro leaves

1. In a small bowl, mix together the coconut aminos, vinegar, and soy sauce.

2. Divide the rice between two plates or bowls. Top each evenly with the greens, carrots, cucumber, mango, avocado (if using), green onions, red onion, and cilantro. Drizzle with the teriyaki coconut aminos or the seasoned rice vinegar and soy sauce.

NUTRITION INFORMATION
SERVING SIZE: 1 serving (not including avocado)   **CALORIES:** 659   **PROTEIN:** 16 g   **CARBS:** 139 g   **FAT:** 2 g

IF ADDING ¼ SMALL AVOCADO, ADD:
CALORIES: 43   **PROTEIN:** 0.5 g   **CARBS:** 0.5 g   **FAT:** 4 g

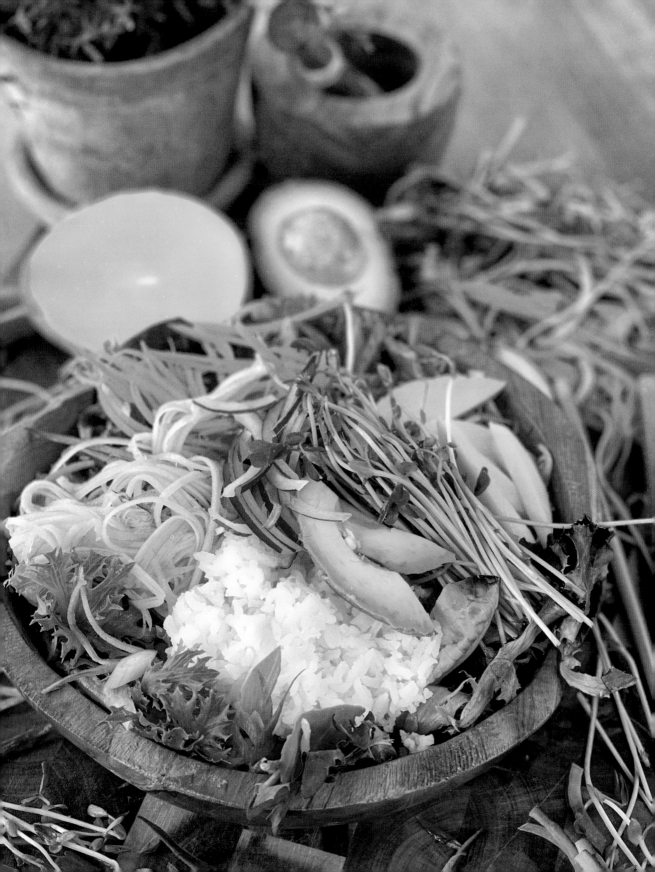

Mediterranean Pasta Salad

SERVES
4

I used to love buying pasta salad from the deli counter at my local grocery store. It was full of mayonnaise and fat and calories… and it was delicious. So naturally, I decided to come up with my own mayonnaise-free version that would be just as delicious but healthy. After some trial and error, I think I've done it. This pasta salad is a terrific potluck option because it's just as good served at room temperature as it is warm. You can also serve it straight from the fridge (see Note).

FOR THE DRESSING

1 (15-ounce) can chickpeas, drained, rinsed, and divided

¼ cup fresh lemon juice

1 tablespoon Dijon mustard

1 tablespoon pure maple syrup

1 teaspoon dried oregano

½ teaspoon garlic powder

½ teaspoon onion powder

½ teaspoon sea salt

Freshly ground black pepper

FOR THE PASTA SALAD

1 (12-ounce) box pasta of your choice (I like Jovial gluten-free brown rice pasta)

2 cups packed fresh spinach

1 cup diced Roma (plum) tomatoes or halved cherry tomatoes

1 cup diced medium English cucumber

1 (2.25-ounce) can pitted black olives, drained and sliced (about ½ cup)

¼ cup diced red onion

¼ cup chopped fresh parsley leaves

Pinch of chili flakes (optional)

1. Bring a large pot of water to a boil for the pasta.

2. **Meanwhile, make the dressing:** In a blender or food processor, combine 1 cup of the chickpeas (reserve the rest for the salad), the lemon juice, mustard, maple syrup, oregano, garlic powder, onion powder, salt, and pepper. Process until smooth and creamy. If the dressing is too thick for your liking, add a little water to thin it out. Set aside.

3. **Make the salad:** When the water comes to a boil, add the pasta and cook according to the package instructions. Drain the pasta, transfer it to a large bowl, and allow it to cool slightly. Add the remaining chickpeas to the bowl, then add the spinach, tomatoes, cucumber, olives, onion, and parsley and toss to combine. Add the dressing and the chili flakes, if desired, and toss to coat well, then serve.

NUTRITION INFORMATION

SERVING SIZE: 2 cups (with whole wheat pasta) **CALORIES:** 450 **PROTEIN:** 11 g **CARBS:** 83 g **FAT:** 5 g

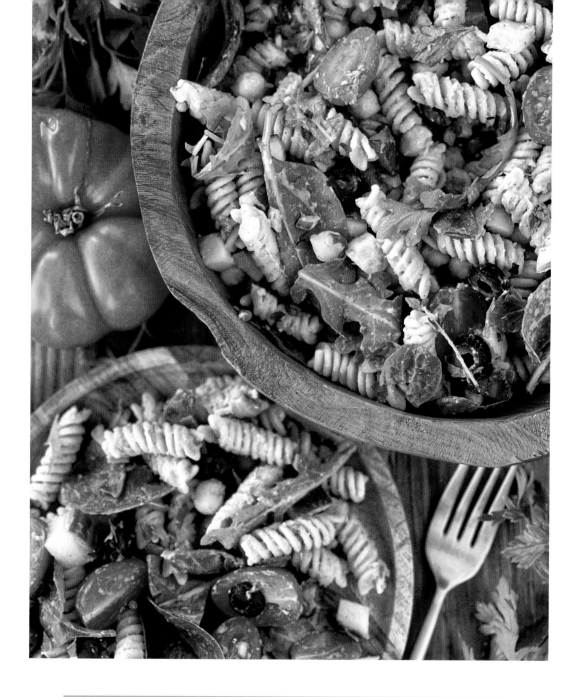

NOTE: If you're using gluten-free pasta, let any leftovers come up to room temperature before serving or pop them in the microwave with a few drops of water for 30 seconds to soften the noodles again.

CHAPTER 3

Soups, Salads, Sides, and Sauces

Tortilla Lime Soup

SERVES
5

When I was growing up, soup was a big deal in my house, and this tortilla soup is hands-down one of my favorites! It's easy to make, inexpensive, and provides plenty of leftovers. I use a low-fat store-bought garlic marinara to flavor this soup. My favorite garlic marinara brands are Sprouts Farmers Market and Whole Foods 365, but use whichever you like. Just look for one with 2.5 g of fat or less per ½ cup.

1 large yellow onion, diced

1 medium jalapeño, seeded and diced

1 (24-ounce) jar low-fat or oil-free garlic marinara sauce

1 (15-ounce) can white beans, such as cannellini or navy, drained and rinsed

1 (15-ounce) can black beans, drained and rinsed

1 (14-ounce) can diced tomatoes, with their juices

1 (14-ounce) can corn kernels, drained and rinsed

½ teaspoon sea salt, plus more as needed

Juice of 1 lime

½ cup chopped fresh cilantro leaves

¼ small avocado, sliced, for serving

2 tablespoons Cashew Sour Cream (page 187), for serving

Baked Corn Tortilla Chips (page 210), for serving

1. In a medium pot, combine the onion and jalapeño. Cook over medium heat until the vegetables are soft, about 3 minutes. Stir in the marinara, beans, tomatoes, corn, and salt. Add 3 cups water and bring the mixture to a boil. Turn off the heat and add the lime juice and cilantro.

2. Ladle into bowls and serve warm, topped with the avocado, sour cream, and tortilla chips.

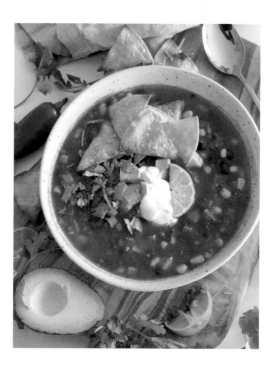

NUTRITION INFORMATION
SERVING SIZE: 2 cups soup with ¼ avocado and 2 tablespoons Cashew Sour Cream   **CALORIES:** 327   **PROTEIN:** 24 g
CARBS: 44 g   **FAT:** 4 g

Spring Ramen Soup

SERVES
2

Everyone loves ramen, right? This ramen delivers big on satisfaction and flavor, and it's so easy to make. The noodles are perfect for slurping, and the garnish of lime and cilantro adds a deep, fresh flavor. The bok choy and mushrooms contribute a nutritional heartiness that makes this soup delicious and filling. The bok choy is loaded with calcium, magnesium, and phosphorus, all of which are excellent for maintaining healthy bones, and the shiitake mushrooms are full of beta-glucans, which help protect against cellular damage and support your immune system.

2 (4-ounce) packages dried Chinese Ramen noodles (I like Ka-Me brand)

10 ounces shiitake mushrooms, sliced

5 vegan chicken-flavor bouillon cubes (I like Edward & Sons Not-Chick'n)

1 pound baby bok choy, ends trimmed

Juice of 1 lime

1 teaspoon chili flakes (optional)

½ cup chopped fresh cilantro leaves

½ cup chopped green onions, white and green parts

1. In a large pot, combine the noodles, mushrooms, 4 bouillon cubes, and 3 cups water. Bring to a boil over medium-high heat and cook until the noodles are soft, 3 to 5 minutes. Turn off the heat. Taste and adjust the seasoning with the remaining bouillon cube, if desired.

2. Add the bok choy and allow it to wilt for 3 minutes before adding the lime juice and chili flakes (if using). Garnish with the cilantro and green onions and serve.

NUTRITION INFORMATION
SERVING SIZE: 1 serving   **CALORIES:** 367   **PROTEIN:** 17 g   **CARBS:** 52 g   **FAT:** 9 g

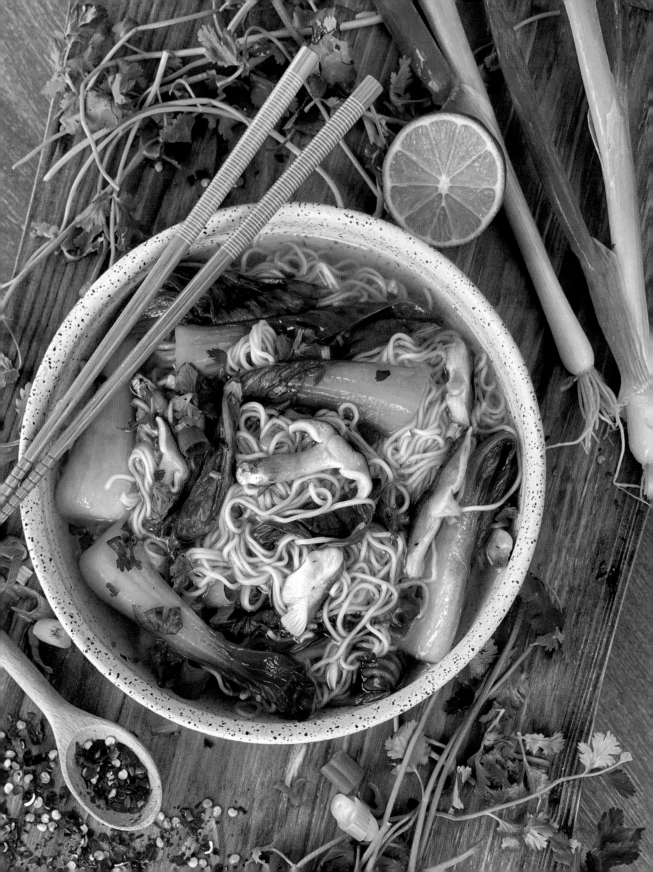

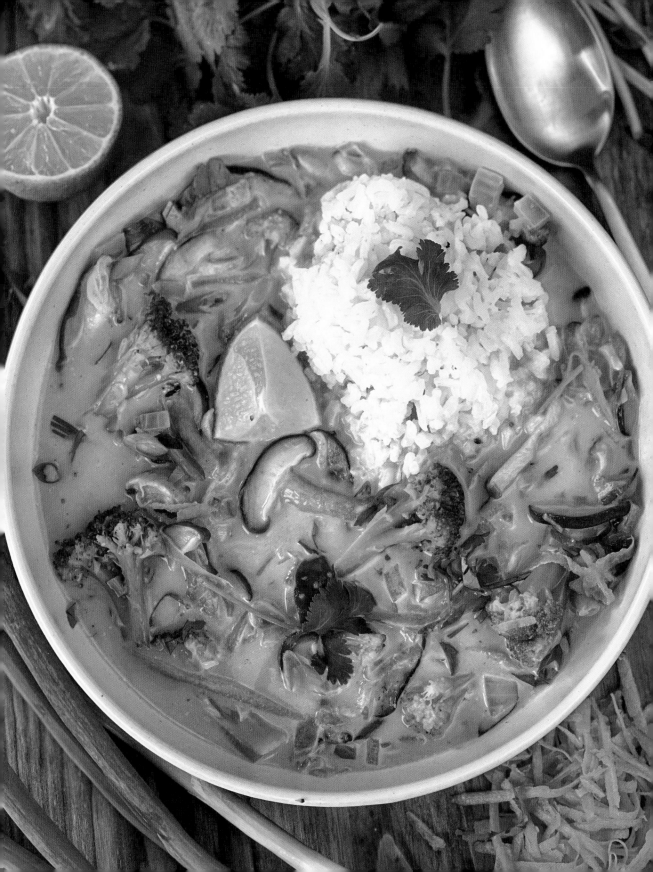

Thai Coconut Curry

Whenever I'm in Breckenridge, Colorado, I make sure to plan a night at an intimate Thai restaurant called Bangkok Happy Bowl, just so I can order their Thai coconut curry. There are yellow curries and red curries, and they're all so creamy and decadent. This is my take on their curry. Even though I'm using light coconut milk, the flavor is all there, and the abundant vegetables (along with fragrant garlic and ginger) make this delicious. Serving the curry over steamed rice takes me back to Bangkok Happy Bowl, no matter where I am.

¾ cup diced yellow onion

1 (14-ounce) can lite coconut milk

5 ounces shiitake mushrooms, sliced

1 cup shredded carrots

1 cup broccoli florets, chopped

2 tablespoons pure maple syrup

1 to 2 tablespoons red curry paste, depending on how spicy you like it

1 tablespoon minced garlic

1 teaspoon minced fresh ginger, or ¼ teaspoon ground ginger

½ teaspoon sea salt, plus more as needed

3 cups white or brown rice, cooked

Juice of ½ lime

¼ cup chopped fresh cilantro leaves

¼ cup sliced green onions, white and green parts

1. In a medium pot, cook the onion over medium-high heat until soft, about 4 minutes. Add the coconut milk, mushrooms, carrots, broccoli, maple syrup, curry paste, garlic, ginger, and salt. Stir in 2 cups water and bring to a boil. Cook for 5 minutes, then turn off the heat.

2. Serve over the rice, garnished with the lime juice, cilantro, and green onions.

NUTRITION INFORMATION
SERVING SIZE: 2 cups curry with 1½ cups steamed rice   **CALORIES:** 592   **PROTEIN:** 12 g   **CARBS:** 98 g   **FAT:** 14 g

Hungarian Mushroom Soup

The sound of "mushroom soup" doesn't seem to excite a lot of people. But this mushroom soup is so full of flavor—with smoked paprika and soy sauce and onions and fresh lemon juice—I promise it will not disappoint. I make this all the time and find that it's especially delicious poured over mashed potatoes! Even my friends and family who swear they don't like mushrooms love this soup.

1 medium yellow onion, diced

16 ounces baby bella (cremini) mushrooms, sliced

1 tablespoon vegetable broth or water

1 vegan chicken-flavor bouillon cube (I like Edward & Sons Not-Chick'n)

1 tablespoon low-sodium soy sauce

1 teaspoon sweet paprika

1 teaspoon smoked paprika

½ teaspoon dried dill

1 cup thick, plain, unsweetened plant-based milk (see headnote on page 97)

¼ cup chopped fresh parsley leaves

2 teaspoons fresh lemon juice

Sea salt and freshly ground black pepper (optional)

1. In a medium pot, combine the onion, mushrooms, and vegetable broth. Cook over medium heat until the vegetables are soft, 6 to 8 minutes. Stir in the bouillon cube, soy sauce, sweet paprika, smoked paprika, and dill. Cover the pot, reduce the heat to low, and simmer for 10 minutes. Turn off the heat.

2. Add the milk, parsley, and lemon juice to the pot and stir to combine. Taste and adjust the seasoning with salt and pepper, if desired. Serve hot.

If you don't *love* mushrooms but are okay with them, or if you enjoy the flavor but can't get past the texture, chop them up instead of leaving them in slices.

NOTE: This soup is very low in calorie density, so do not rely on it as a main source of calories. Use it as an appetizer or enjoy it as the vegetable side to a plate.

NUTRITION INFORMATION
SERVING SIZE: 2 cups CALORIES: 123 PROTEIN: 10 g CARBS: 10 g FAT: 4 g

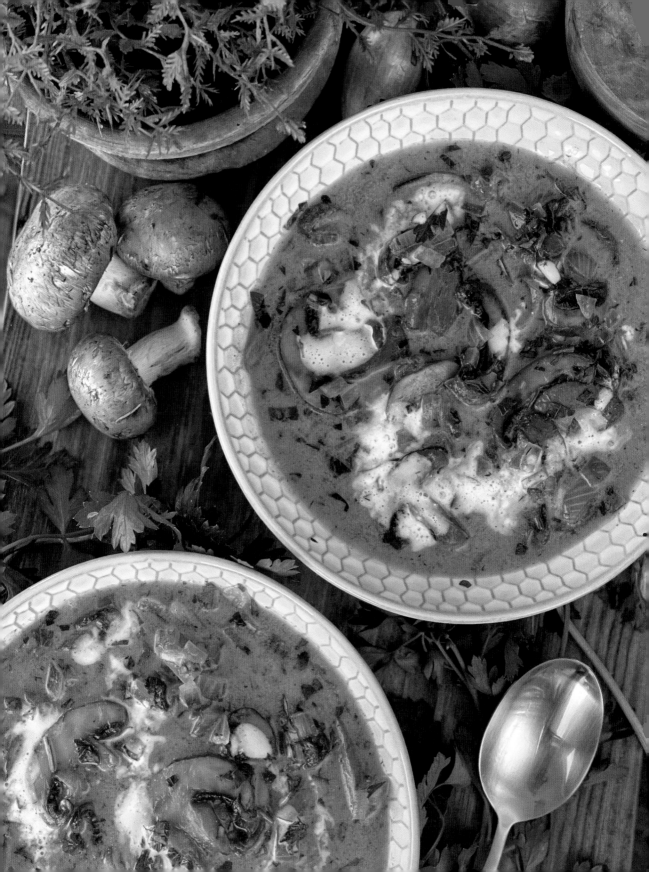

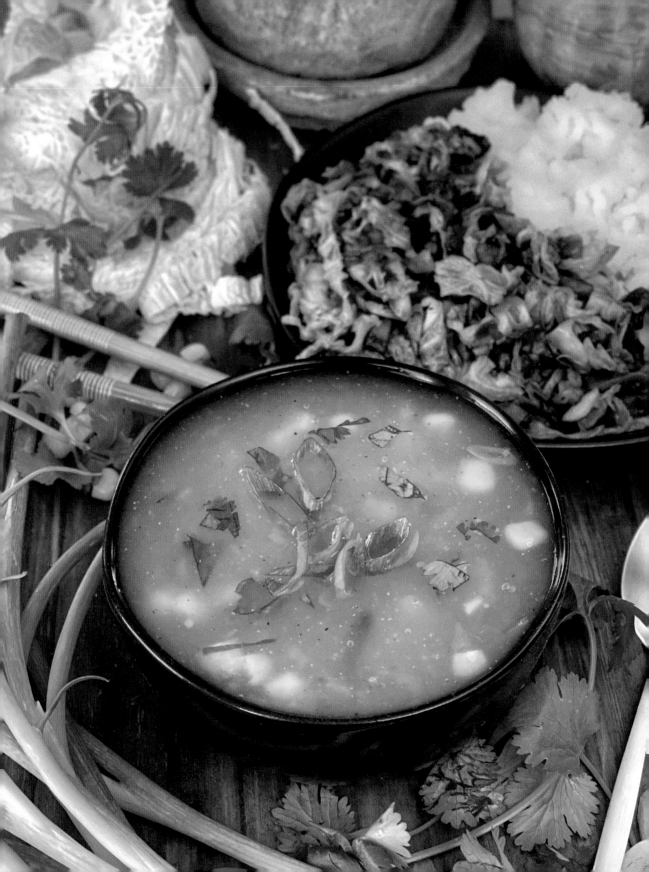

Eggless Egg Drop Soup

SERVES
2

I know it's old-school, but one of the things I love about our local Chinese restaurant's takeout menus is being faced with the happy choice of egg drop soup or sweet-and-sour soup. I love both, but wanted the challenge of coming up with a vegan egg drop number. I think this version really does taste like the original. Just that little bit of toasted sesame oil gives it the familiar, authentic flavor.

2 chicken-flavor vegan bouillon cubes
(I like Edward & Sons Not-Chick'n)

¼ teaspoon garlic powder or ½ teaspoon minced
fresh garlic

Pinch of ground turmeric (optional, for color)

¼ cup plus 2 tablespoons cornstarch

½ cup fresh or canned corn kernels
(drained, if canned)

¼ cup plus 2 tablespoons minced green onions,
white and green parts

½ teaspoon toasted sesame oil (optional; see Note)

Freshly ground black pepper

1. In a medium pot, combine the bouillon cubes, garlic powder, turmeric (if using), and 4 cups water. Bring to a boil over medium-high heat.

2. In a small bowl, mix together the cornstarch and ½ cup cold water. Stir the mixture into the boiling broth. Reduce the heat to maintain a simmer and cook for 1 minute, until the broth thickens. Turn off the heat and stir in the corn, green onions, sesame oil (if using), and pepper to taste. Divide between two small bowls and serve hot.

NOTE: This soup is very low in calorie density, so do not rely on it as a main source of calories. Use it as an appetizer or as a side to your meal. If you include the toasted sesame oil, add 20 calories and 2 grams of fat to the nutritional totals.

NUTRITION INFORMATION
SERVING SIZE: 1 serving **CALORIES:** 164 **PROTEIN:** 2 g **CARBS:** 28 g **FAT:** 5 g

French Onion Soup

SERVES
2

My mom and I share a love of soup, and French onion is one of her favorites. I wanted to find a way to make a low-calorie plant-based version, so I set out to see if this soup would still satisfy without all the cheese that normally tops it—and it does! When you add the toasted bread with cheese sauce, this becomes a comforting soup.

2 large Vidalia onions, sliced

1 tablespoon minced garlic

2 dried bay leaves

¼ teaspoon herbes de Provence or dried thyme

½ cup red wine

**2 vegan chicken-flavor bouillon cubes
(I like Edward & Sons Not-Chick'n)**

Sea salt and freshly ground black pepper

2 slices bread of your choice, toasted

**½ cup Cheese Sauce (page 176), for serving
(see Note)**

Fresh thyme leaves, for garnish

1. In a medium pot, combine the onions, garlic, bay leaves, and herbes de Provence. Cook over medium heat, stirring occasionally, until the onions are soft, about 15 minutes. If the pan gets dry, add a splash of water.

2. Stir in the wine and bring the mixture to a simmer, then cook for 5 minutes to allow the alcohol to cook off. Remove the bay leaves and discard. Add the bouillon cubes and 4 cups water and whisk until the bouillon cubes have dissolved. Taste and adjust the seasoning with salt and pepper, if needed.

3. Transfer the soup to bowls and top each with a piece of toast. Drizzle with the cheese sauce, garnish with parsley, and serve.

NOTE: This soup is very low in calorie density, so do not rely on it as a main source of calories. Use it as an appetizer or as a side to your meal. If you'd like to make the cheese sauce white in order to make this look more like the original, just omit the carrots.

NUTRITION INFORMATION
SERVING SIZE: 2 cups soup with 1 slice sprouted whole-grain bread and ¼ cup Cheese Sauce   **CALORIES:** 240
PROTEIN: 8 g   **CARBS:** 33 g   **FAT:** 5 g
SERVING SIZE: 2 cups soup (without bread or Cheese Sauce)   **CALORIES:** 104   **PROTEIN:** 3 g   **CARBS:** 13 g   **FAT:** 3 g

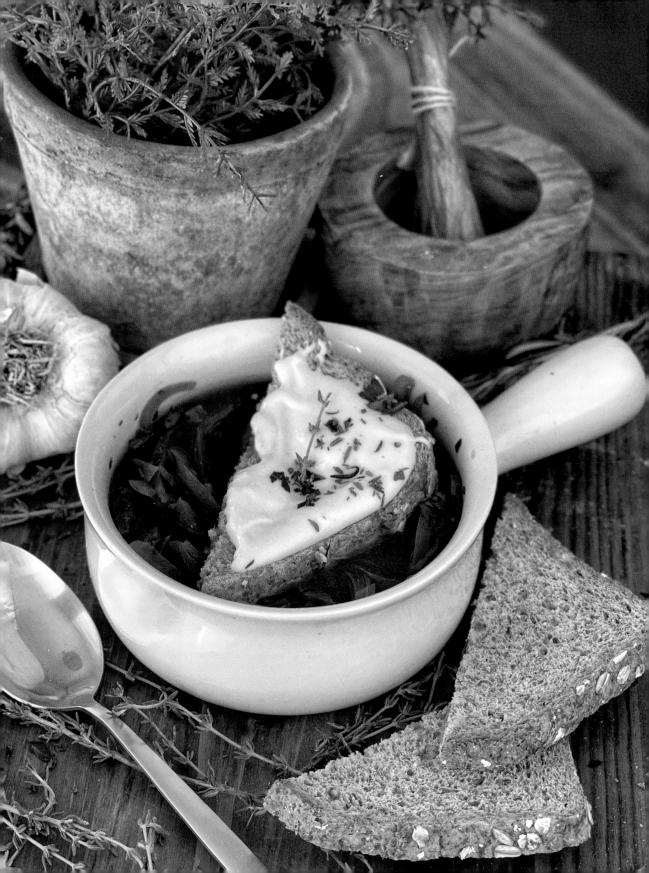

Creamy Poblano Soup

SERVES
2

Creamy potato soups are one of my absolute favorite soup subcategories. This one is smooth and decadent without all the fat and calories you'd get in the standard version. In Colorado, our weekly farmers' markets are filled with the aroma of fire-roasted poblano peppers, which I've added to this soup to give it a smoky, earthy flavor that melts in your mouth when combined with the creaminess of the soup. What's unique about this soup is that it makes a great summer and winter soup!

---

3 poblano peppers (see Note)

1½ large russet potatoes, peeled and diced

½ cup raw unsalted cashews (optional; see Note)

2 teaspoons fresh lemon juice

2 teaspoons garlic powder or minced fresh garlic

2 teaspoons sea salt

1 teaspoon onion powder

1 medium yellow onion, diced

½ cup canned or fresh corn kernels (drained, if canned)

½ cup chopped fresh cilantro leaves

---

1. Preheat the oven to 450°F. Line a baking sheet with parchment paper.

2. Set the peppers on the prepared baking sheet and roast for 40 minutes, or until very soft. (Alternatively, cook them in an air fryer for 30 minutes.) Transfer the peppers to a bowl or container and cover with plastic wrap or a lid; let stand for 10 minutes. When just cool enough to handle, gently peel the skins from the peppers and discard. Remove the stems. If you want less heat, remove the seeds and discard. Roughly chop the peppers and set aside.

3. Meanwhile, place the potatoes in a small pot and add enough cold water to just cover them. Bring to a boil, reduce the heat to maintain a simmer, and cook until the potatoes are easily pierced by a fork, about 15 minutes. Drain the potatoes in a colander set over a large bowl and let cool slightly; reserve the cooking water.

4. Coarsely chop the potatoes and transfer them to a blender. Add the cashews (if using), lemon juice, garlic powder, salt, onion powder, and 2 cups of the reserved cooking water and blend until smooth. Add more of the reserved cooking water to adjust the consistency of the soup to your liking.

5. In a large nonstick sauté pan, cook the onion over medium heat, stirring occasionally, until soft, about 5 minutes. Add the blended soup and stir in the corn, roasted peppers, and cilantro. Divide between two bowls and serve hot.

NUTRITION INFORMATION
SERVING SIZE: 2½ cups (made with ½ cup cashews)   **CALORIES:** 559   **PROTEIN:** 15 g   **CARBS:** 84 g   **FAT:** 15 g

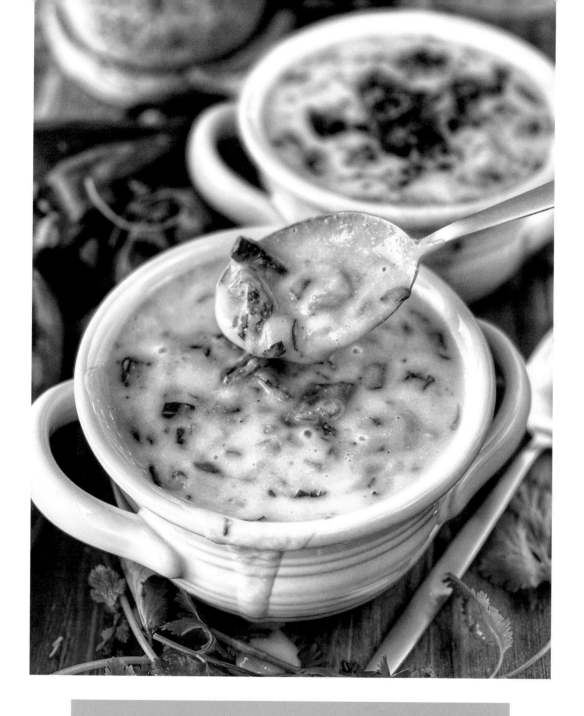

NOTE: I call for roasting the poblano peppers yourself, but you could also buy canned or jarred ones and use ½ cup. To reduce the calories and fat in this recipe, you can reduce the cashews to ¼ cup or omit them altogether. For a nut-free substitute, use hemp hearts.

House Salad

This really is my house salad—I make it several times a week. We always have the few ingredients required, and when dressed with my ranch, it's satisfying and nutritious. If you have carrots, tomatoes, greens, and onions on your shopping list every week and keep them cleaned and prepped in the fridge, you'll be able to pull together this salad without even thinking about it.

Put the greens in a large bowl and top with the tomatoes, cucumber, carrots, and onion. Give everything a toss, then drizzle with the dressing. Toss again to coat and serve.

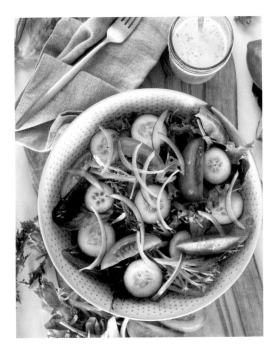

8 cups spring greens or chopped romaine lettuce

1 cup sliced cherry tomatoes or diced Roma (plum) tomatoes

1 medium English cucumber, sliced

½ cup shredded carrots

¼ cup thinly sliced red onion

½ cup Cashew Ranch Dressing (page 181)

NUTRITION INFORMATION
SERVING SIZE: 1 serving   **CALORIES:** 139   **PROTEIN:** 7 g   **CARBS:** 13 g   **FAT:** 7 g

Caesar Salad

My creamy Caesar dressing makes this tasty, but don't skip the croutons! I feel like a Caesar salad isn't a Caesar salad without the crunch of the croutons. Don't forget to season the salad with a little extra salt and pepper. If you're really missing the parmesan, try shaving some vegan parm over the salad—I like Violife's parmesan-style wedge, which adds lots of flavor but only minimal calories.

2 slices sprouted whole-grain bread or gluten-free bread, cut into ½-inch cubes

¼ teaspoon garlic powder

¼ teaspoon sea salt, plus more as needed

8 cups chopped romaine lettuce

¼ small red onion, thinly sliced

½ cup Caesar Dressing (page 175)

Freshly ground black pepper

Vegan parmesan cheese (I like Violife), for serving (optional)

1. Preheat the oven or air fryer to 400°F. Spread the bread cubes evenly over a baking sheet or the basket of your air fryer. Season with the garlic powder and salt and bake or air-fry for 3 to 5 minutes, until golden brown.

2. Put the lettuce in a large bowl and top with the croutons, onion, and dressing. Toss and season with more salt, if needed, and some pepper. Grate some vegan parm over the top, if desired, and serve.

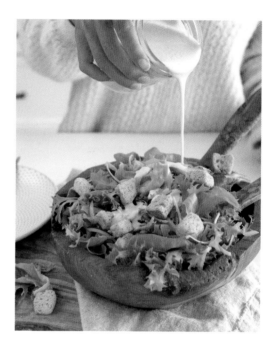

NUTRITION INFORMATION
SERVING SIZE: 1 serving (not including vegan parmesan)   **CALORIES:** 216   **PROTEIN:** 11 g   **CARBS:** 22 g   **FAT:** 7 g

Thai-Inspired Noodle Salad

SERVES
2

The smaller you dice the vegetables and the finer you slice the greens and cabbage in this Thai-inspired salad, the more enjoyable it is, because the dressing coats everything more evenly. I use a grater or food processor to shred the carrots and chop the cilantro and Thai basil.

FOR THE SALAD
4 ounces dried soba noodles

8 cups thinly sliced red-leaf lettuce

2 cups thinly sliced lacinato kale leaves
(ribs removed)

1 cup thinly sliced red cabbage

½ cup finely diced red bell pepper

1 cup sliced cucumber

4 green onions, white and green parts sliced

1 cup shredded carrots

1 cup fresh cilantro, chopped

6 fresh Thai basil leaves, chopped into small pieces

1 cup fresh or canned mandarin orange segments (if
using canned, drain segments)

FOR THE SPICY THAI PEANUT SAUCE
½ cup powdered peanut butter, such as PB2

4 tablespoons low-sodium soy sauce

2 teaspoon toasted sesame oil

1 teaspoon ginger paste, store-bought

4 teaspoons oil-free chili paste (I like sambal oelek)

10 drops stevia, or more to taste

1. **Make the salad:** Bring a large pot of water to a boil and cook the soba noodles according to the package instructions. Drain and rinse the noodles and set aside to cool slightly.

2. In a medium bowl, combine the lettuce, kale, cabbage, bell pepper, cucumber, green onions, carrots, cilantro, and basil.

3. **Make the sauce:** In a small bowl, whisk together the peanut butter powder, soy sauce, sesame oil, ginger paste, chili paste, stevia, and 3 tablespoons water until smooth.

4. Add the noodles to the bowl with the greens and veggies and mix well, then add the sauce and toss to coat. Top with the mandarin oranges and enjoy.

NUTRITION INFORMATION
SERVING SIZE: 1 serving   CALORIES: 506   PROTEIN: 27 g   CARBS: 77 g   FAT: 9 g

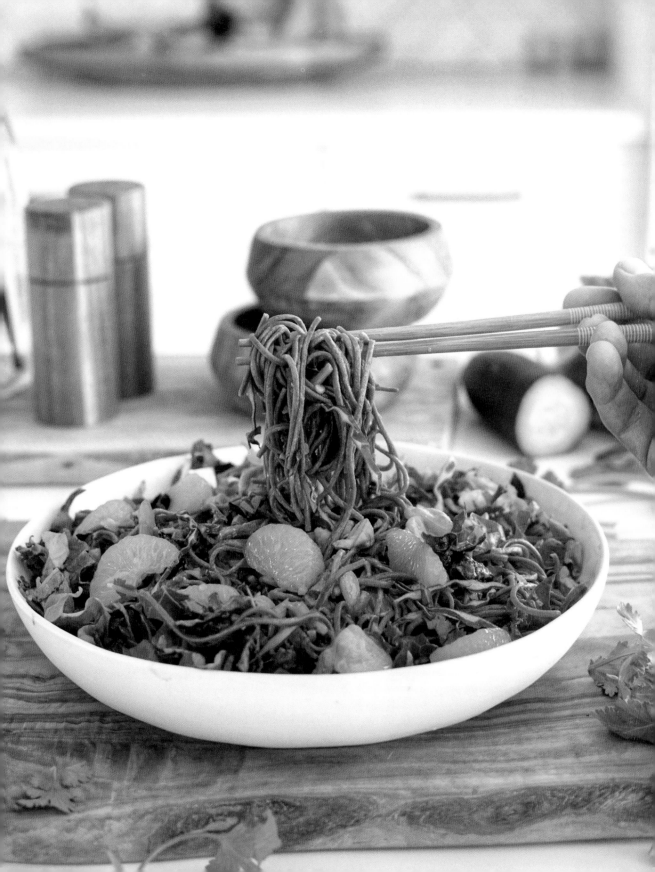

Southwest Salad

SERVES
2

I love this dish because you can serve it as is for a tasty salad full of greens and veggies, or add beans and rice to make it a filling meal. The Southwest Ranch tops it off perfectly.

---

8 cups spring greens or chopped romaine lettuce

1 medium English cucumber, sliced

1 cup sliced cherry tomatoes or diced Roma (plum) tomatoes

½ cup shredded carrots

¼ cup thinly sliced red onion

¼ cup canned or fresh corn kernels (drained, if canned)

1 medium jalapeño, seeded and sliced (optional)

½ cup canned black beans, drained and rinsed (optional)

1 cup white or brown rice, cooked, for serving (optional; see Note)

½ small avocado, sliced (optional)

½ cup Southwest Ranch (page 179)

1. Place the greens in a large bowl and top with the cucumber, tomatoes, carrots, onion, corn, and jalapeño (if using). Give everything a toss to combine.

2. Add the beans, rice, and/or avocado, if desired. Drizzle the dressing over the salad and serve.

> **NOTE:** Adding white or brown rice to this recipe makes it a ⁵⁰/₅₀ meal; just adjust the nutrition info accordingly. Similarly, you can add beans and/or avocado to make this an even heartier salad. Again, the adjusted nutrition info is below.

NUTRITION INFORMATION
SERVING SIZE: 1 serving (not including beans, avocado, or rice)   **CALORIES:** 191   **PROTEIN:** 11 g   **CARBS:** 23 g   **FAT:** 6 g
SERVING SIZE: 1 serving, with beans and avocado (no rice)   **CALORIES:** 291   **PROTEIN:** 13 g   **CARBS:** 28 g   **FAT:** 12 g
SERVING SIZE: 1 serving, with beans, avocado, and rice   **CALORIES:** 497   **PROTEIN:** 17 g   **CARBS:** 72 g   **FAT:** 12 g

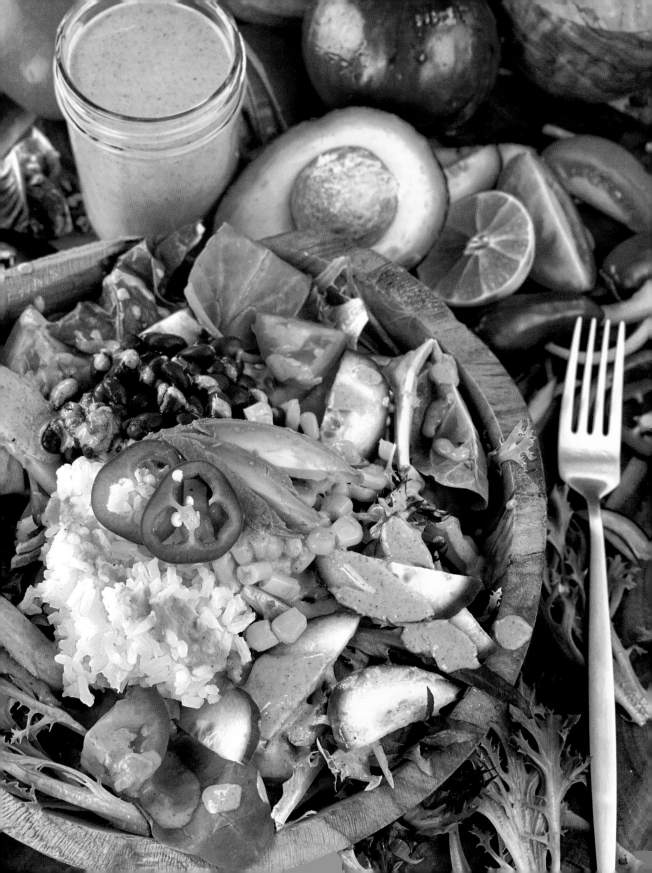

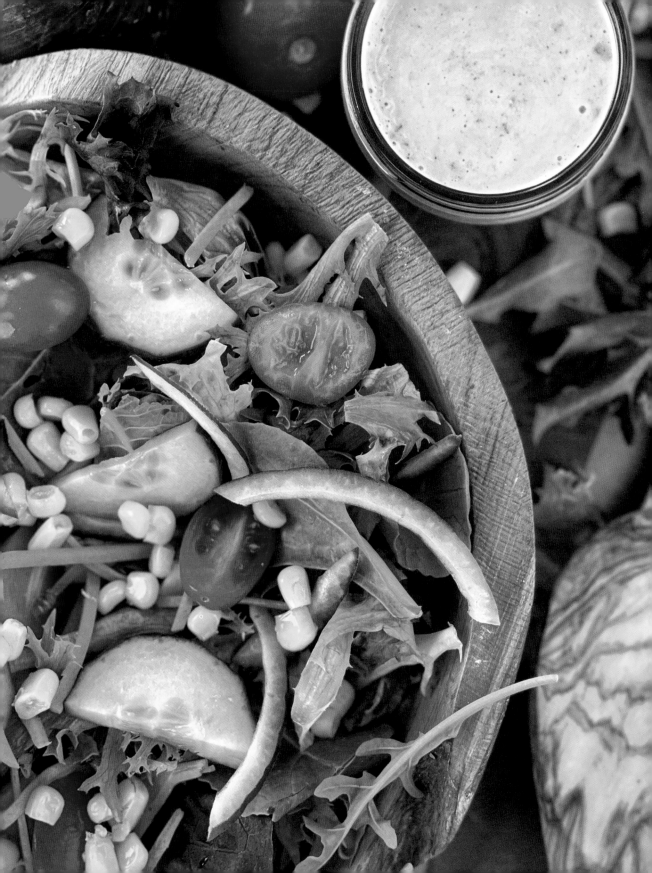

BBQ Salad

SERVES
2

Since this is such a simple salad that can be prepped ahead of time, I find it goes best with my Smokehouse Steak Fries (page 94). You can even throw your fries into the salad for a delicious and filling bowl!

8 cups spring greens or chopped romaine lettuce

1 medium English cucumber, sliced

1 cup sliced cherry tomatoes or diced Roma (plum) tomatoes

½ cup shredded carrots

½ cup canned or fresh corn kernels (drained, if canned)

¼ cup thinly sliced red onion

½ cup BBQ Ranch (page 178)

Put the greens in a large bowl and top with the cucumber, tomatoes, carrots, corn, and onion. Drizzle with the dressing and serve.

NUTRITION INFORMATION
SERVING SIZE: 1 serving   CALORIES: 198   PROTEIN: 8 g   CARBS: 25 g   FAT: 6 g

Buffalo Cauliflower Wing Salad

Friday nights are for either pizza or wings in our house! When we transitioned to a plant-based diet, I missed those treats and was craving that fun "weekend food." Then I started making this cauliflower. With the delicious Buffalo dressing and crispy baked bread crumb coating, it really is a whole meal—one that I love and that my family enjoys equally.

---

2 medium heads cauliflower, chopped into florets

1½ cups panko bread crumbs or gluten-free bread crumbs

¾ cup low-fat or fat-free wing sauce (I like Frank's RedHot in mild)

8 cups spring greens

1 cup diced tomatoes

1 cup sliced cucumber

⅔ cup sliced or diced red onion

¾ cup Cashew Ranch Dressing (page 181)

---

1. Preheat the oven or air fryer to 425°F. Line a baking sheet with parchment paper.

2. In a large bowl, combine the cauliflower, panko, and wing sauce. Toss to mix well. Spread the mixture over the prepared baking sheet or the basket of the air fryer. Bake or air-fry for 20 minutes, or until the cauliflower is crispy.

3. Put the greens in a separate large bowl and top with the tomatoes, cucumber, onion, and crispy cauliflower. Drizzle with the dressing and serve.

NUTRITION INFORMATION
SERVING SIZE: 1 serving   **CALORIES:** 550   **PROTEIN:** 27 g   **CARBS:** 62 g   **FAT:** 17 g

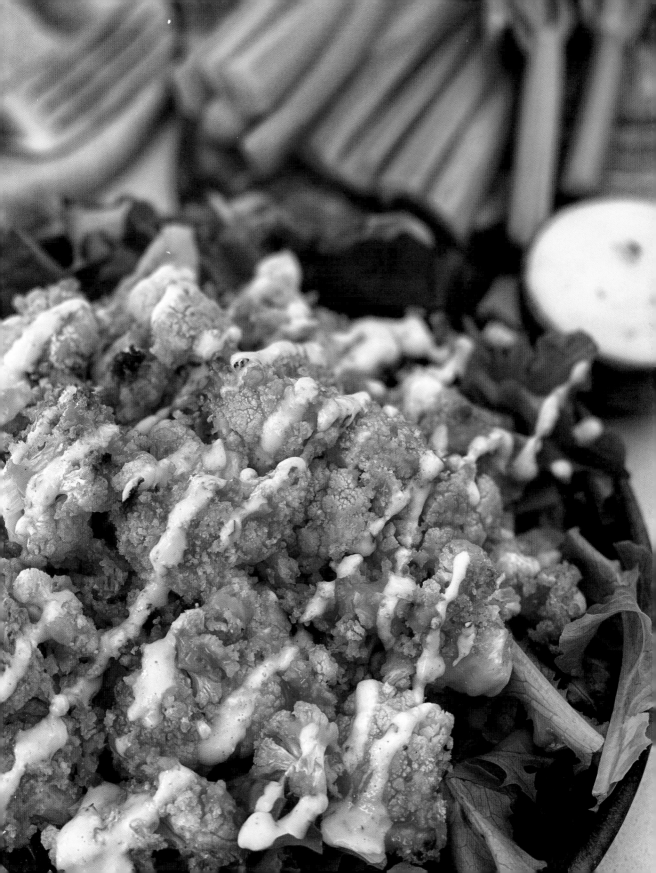

Cucumber Salad

When you want something fresh and crunchy, this cucumber salad hits the spot. This is a go-to for me in the summer when barbecue season starts. Because it's so simple to put together, travels well, and is always a crowd-pleaser, I take it to just about every gathering. I love pairing this with sushi as my vegetable side.

Use a vegetable peeler, mandoline, or sharp knife to cut the cucumbers into thin strips. Put the cucumber strips in a large bowl and add the carrots, green onions, rice vinegar, and maple syrup (if using). Toss to combine, garnish with a sprinkling of sesame seeds, and serve.

4 medium English cucumbers

2 medium carrots, shredded

2 green onions, white and green parts sliced

¼ cup seasoned rice vinegar

2 teaspoons pure maple syrup (optional)

Sesame seeds, for garnish

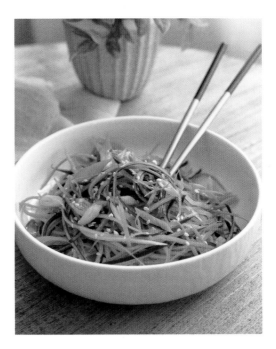

NUTRITION INFORMATION

SERVING SIZE: 1 serving **CALORIES:** 162 **PROTEIN:** 4 g **CARBS:** 31 g **FAT:** 1 g

Steamed or Roasted Asparagus

SERVES
1 OR 2

There are three keys to tasty vegetables: cooking them perfectly, the seasoning, and the dressing. Whether I steam or roast my asparagus, garlic salt is a must for me, and I especially love asparagus with my Maple Mustard Dressing.

---

1 pound asparagus, trimmed

SERVING OPTIONS
⅛ **teaspoon garlic salt**
1 tablespoon coconut aminos teriyaki sauce (I like Coconut Secret)
1 tablespoon Maple Mustard Dressing (page 184)
1 tablespoon aged balsamic vinegar

---

1. *If roasting the asparagus,* preheat the oven to 425°F. Line a baking sheet with parchment paper.

2. Arrange the asparagus on the prepared baking sheet in a single layer and roast for 10 minutes, or until tender but not soft. Remove from the oven and serve—I love this version seasoned with garlic salt.

3. *If steaming the asparagus,* fill a large pot with a fitted lid with 2 inches of water. Bring the water up to a simmer. Put the asparagus in a steamer basket and place it in the pot. Cover the pot and steam for 3 minutes, until the asparagus is tender but not soft. Remove the asparagus from the steamer and top with the teriyaki sauce, maple mustard dressing, balsamic vinegar, or any other seasoning options.

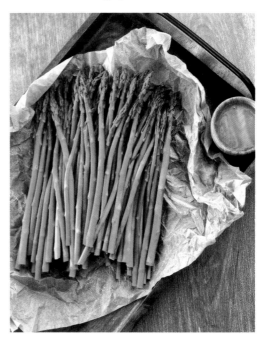

NUTRITION INFORMATION
SERVING SIZE: 1 serving with 1 tablespoon coconut aminos teriyaki sauce   **CALORIES:** 76   **PROTEIN:** 6 g   **CARBS:** 12 g   **FAT:** 1 g

Smoky Apple and Greens Salad

This is a great fall and winter salad. Sweet and juicy apples pair so well with fresh cucumber, and the smoky variation of my Maple Mustard Dressing makes the perfect combination.

8 cups spring greens or romaine lettuce
1 medium English cucumber, sliced
1 Honeycrisp apple, cored and sliced
¼ cup thinly sliced red onion
¼ cup Smoky Maple Mustard Dressing
(see page 184)

In a large bowl, combine the greens, cucumber, apple, onion, and dressing. Toss to coat well and serve.

NUTRITION INFORMATION
SERVING SIZE: 1 serving   **CALORIES:** 158   **PROTEIN:** 4 g   **CARBS:** 31 g   **FAT:** 1 g

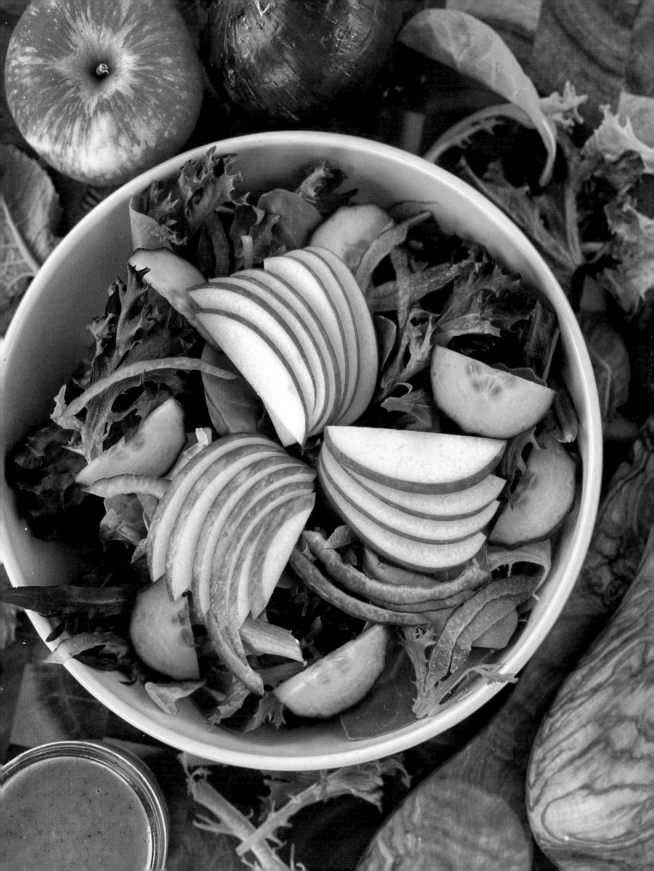

Roasted Brussels Sprout and Mushroom Mix

Roasted Brussels sprouts are a revelation! They're crispy and tender and, depending on how you season them, full of satisfying flavor. I like to toss mine in a good balsamic vinegar and season them with garlic salt before I roast them. I also like to give them a light spray of avocado oil to help them crisp up.

1 pound Brussels sprouts, ends trimmed and halved lengthwise (or quartered, if large)

16 ounces baby bella (cremini) or white mushrooms, halved (see Note)

1 medium Vidalia onion, sliced (see Note)

2 tablespoons aged balsamic vinegar, for serving (optional)

¼ teaspoon garlic salt

Avocado oil cooking spray

2 tablespoons Maple Mustard Dressing (page 184), for serving (optional)

1. Preheat the oven to 425°F. Line a baking sheet with parchment paper.

2. Arrange the Brussels sprouts, mushrooms, and onion in a single layer on the prepared baking sheet. Sprinkle them with the vinegar and season with the garlic salt. Toss well to coat. Lightly spray with avocado oil and roast for 20 to 30 minutes, until tender and crisp.

3. Drizzle with the dressing or additional vinegar, if desired, and serve.

NOTE: Another tasty variation is to toss the Brussels sprouts with 2 tablespoons soy sauce and the garlic salt before roasting. And if you're pressed for time, you can skip the mushrooms and onions.

NUTRITIONAL INFORMATION
SERVING SIZE: 1 serving with 1 tablespoon dressing **CALORIES:** 243 **PROTEIN:** 1 g **CARBS:** 34 g **FAT:** 2 g

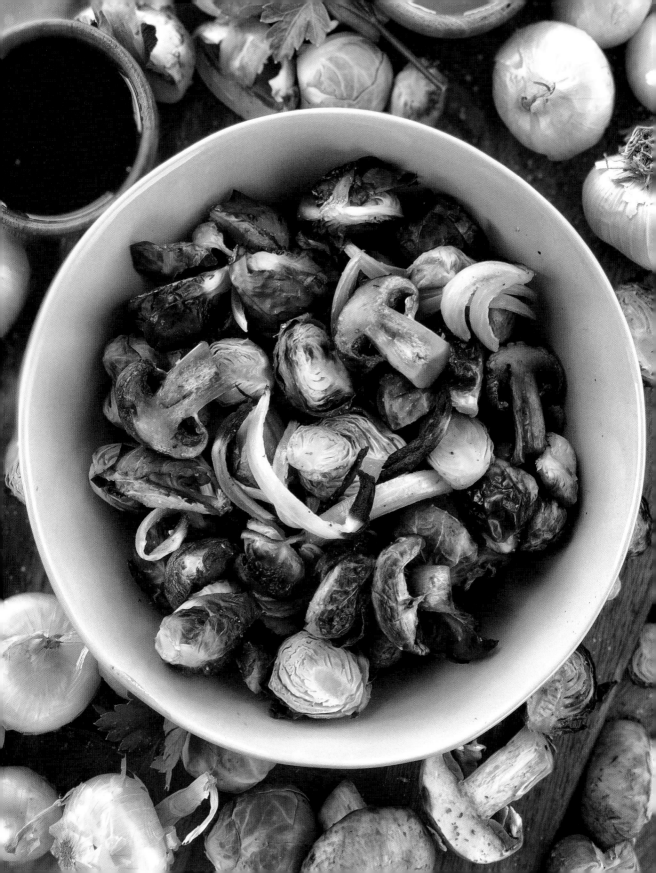

Steamed Broccoli with Cheese Sauce

When I was growing up, my mom would entice my brother and me to eat broccoli by covering it in that melty processed cheese product that most of us know and loved. So as an adult, naturally I want cheese sauce on my broccoli—but a more grown-up, cheese-forward version, not the stuff from a can. That's where my delicious cheese sauce comes into play. You can really eat an entire bowl of steamed broccoli when it's covered in whole food cheese sauce!

1 pound fresh or frozen broccoli florets
¼ teaspoon garlic powder or minced fresh garlic
Sea salt to taste
Freshly ground black pepper
½ cup Cheese Sauce (page 176)

1. Fill a medium pot with a fitted lid with 2 inches of water and bring to a simmer over medium heat. Put the broccoli in a steamer basket and place it in the pot. Cover the pot and steam for 5 to 10 minutes, until the broccoli is bright green and tender but not mushy. (Alternatively, put the broccoli in a microwave-safe container, add 1 tablespoon water, cover, and microwave on high for 2 to 4 minutes or until fork tender.)

2. Season the broccoli with the garlic salt and pepper to taste and serve smothered with the cheese sauce.

NUTRITION INFORMATION
SERVING SIZE: 1 serving   **CALORIES:** 120   **PROTEIN:** 9 g   **CARBS:** 14 g   **FAT:** 2 g

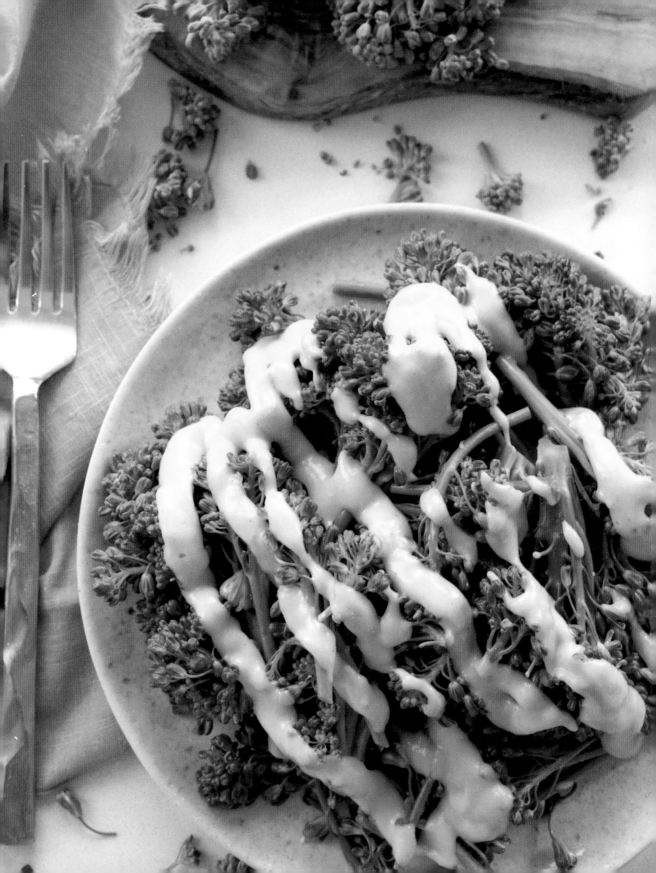

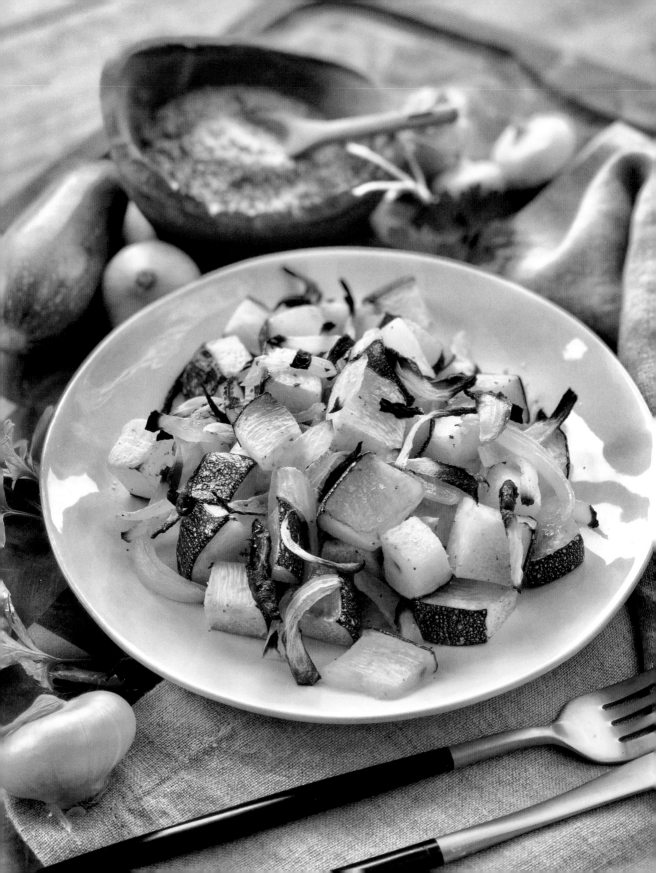

Garlic Roasted
Zucchini and Onion

Every summer we seem to have an abundance of both zucchini and onions from our garden. We love roasting them together, because the onion caramelizes and adds a delicious, sweet flavor to this simple garden combo. My favorite way to season this is with garlic salt and a light spray of oil before roasting—that's it!

1. Preheat the oven to 425°F. Line a baking sheet with parchment paper.

2. Arrange the vegetables in a single layer on the prepared baking sheet. Lightly spray them with the avocado oil and toss with the garlic salt and rosemary. Roast for 20 to 30 minutes, until the vegetables are beginning to brown. Season with more garlic salt, if desired, and serve.

4 cups chopped zucchini
1 medium Vidalia onion, sliced
Avocado oil cooking spray
¼ teaspoon garlic salt, plus more as needed
Pinch of dried rosemary

> **NOTE:** For other delicious variations of this dish, try tossing the vegetables with 1 tablespoon coconut aminos teriyaki sauce (I like Coconut Secret), 1 tablespoon aged balsamic vinegar, or 1 tablespoon soy sauce along with the garlic salt before roasting.

NUTRITION INFORMATION
SERVING SIZE: 1 serving   **CALORIES:** 145   **PROTEIN:** 8 g   **CARBS:** 21 g   **FAT:** 2 g

Stir-Fry Mix

SERVES
1 OR 2

Whether you buy premixed bags of stir-fry vegetables or assemble your own combination, a stir-fry comes down to the sauce. My favorite way to eat these steamed veggies is with my Sweet Soy Ginger Sauce or some coconut aminos teriyaki sauce, because it's simple, sweet, and tangy.

1 small red onion, sliced

1 cup fresh broccoli florets

1 cup baby bella (cremini) mushrooms, quartered

½ cup snow peas

½ cup green beans, trimmed

1 red bell pepper, sliced

1 tablespoon water chestnuts, drained

OPTIONAL SAUCE ADD-IN

2 tablespoons low-sodium soy sauce

2 tablespoons store-bought sweet chili sauce

2 tablespoons Sweet Soy Ginger Sauce (page 185)

2 tablespoons teriyaki coconut aminos
(I like Coconut Secret)

In a large nonstick sauté pan, combine the onions, broccoli, mushrooms, snow peas, green beans, bell pepper, and water chestnuts. Stir in the sauce of your choice and toss to combine. Cook over medium heat, stirring occasionally, until the vegetables are tender, 8 to 10 minutes.

NOTE: You can use 1 (16-ounce) bag of frozen mixed stir-fry vegetables in place of the fresh vegetables.

NUTRITION INFORMATION
SERVING SIZE: 1 serving with 2 tablespoons soy sauce **CALORIES:** 165 **PROTEIN:** 11 g **CARBS:** 23 g **FAT:** 2 g

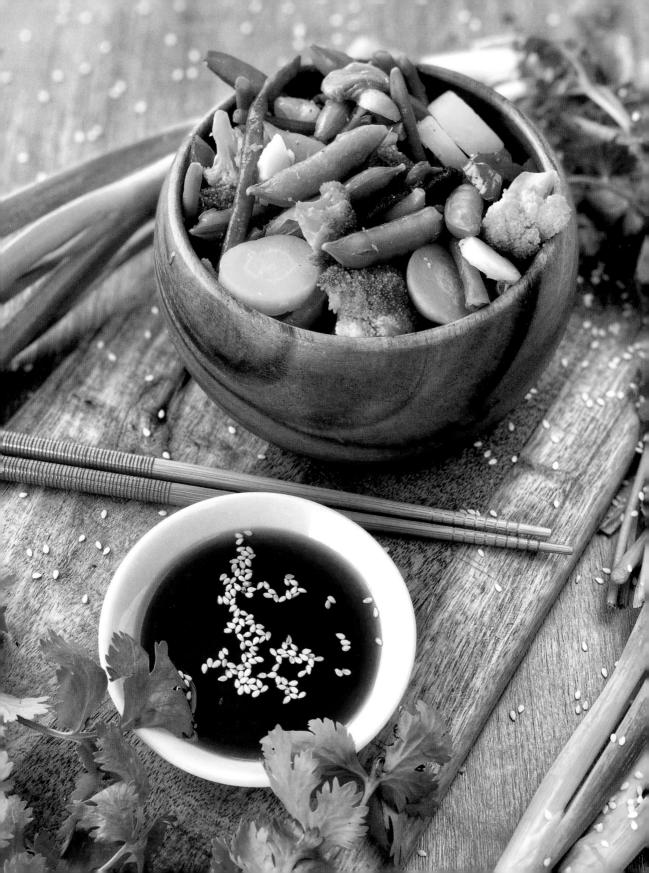

Turmeric-Roasted Cauliflower

I was at a friend's house for dinner when she announced that she had made me a large pan of roasted cauliflower because she knows I'm a plant-based eater. I smiled and thanked her politely as best I could, because the truth is, I'm not crazy about cauliflower. But when I tried her cauliflower, my jaw dropped! What I learned that day is that there are three keys to good roasted cauliflower: one, a spray of oil so it roasts well; two, seasoning it well with garlic salt; and three, letting it roast until it has browned—even to the verge of very brown—for more flavor and texture. The combination of the garlic salt, turmeric, and caraway seeds is phenomenal!

---

1 medium head cauliflower, chopped into bite-size pieces

3 tablespoons vegetable broth or fresh lemon juice (optional)

Avocado oil cooking spray (optional)

¼ teaspoon ground turmeric

¼ teaspoon garlic salt

¼ teaspoon caraway seeds

---

1. Preheat the oven to 425°F. Line a baking sheet with parchment paper.

2. Spread the cauliflower over the prepared baking sheet. Sprinkle with the broth or lightly spray it with avocado oil. Season with the turmeric, garlic salt, and caraway seeds and toss to coat well. Roast for 20 to 30 minutes, until the cauliflower is tender and crispy. Serve immediately.

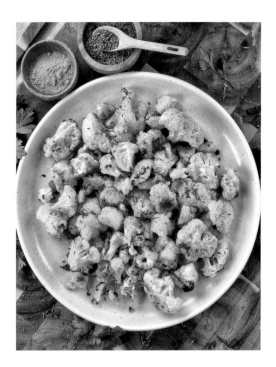

NUTRITION INFORMATION
SERVING SIZE: 1 serving   **CALORIES:** 154   **PROTEIN:** 12 g   **CARBS:** 18 g   **FAT:** 2 g

Roasted Cauliflower Steaks with Pesto

I had the most amazing roasted cauliflower with pesto at a cute little Italian restaurant in San Diego. Naturally, I wanted to make my own version that would be low in fat and calories. This one is simple and wholesome, and if you have leftover pesto, you can save it for pasta. Just store it in an airtight container in the fridge for up to five days.

3. Meanwhile, in a blender, combine the beans, basil, lemon juice, nutritional yeast (if using), garlic salt, and pepper. Blend until smooth. Taste and adjust the seasoning with more garlic salt and pepper, if needed.

4. Divide pesto evenly over the steaks and enjoy.

1 medium head cauliflower, sliced through the stem end into ½-inch-thick steaks

½ (15-ounce) can white cannellini beans, drained and rinsed

¼ cup packed fresh basil leaves

Juice of ¼ lemon

1½ teaspoons nutritional yeast (optional)

¼ teaspoon garlic salt, plus more as needed

Freshly ground black pepper

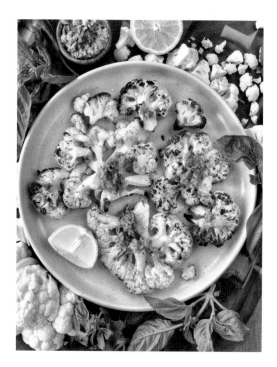

1. Preheat the oven to 425°F. Line a baking sheet with parchment paper.

2. Arrange the cauliflower steaks in a single layer on the prepared baking sheet. Sprinkle each steak on both sides with the garlic salt. Roast for 20 to 30 minutes, until just starting to brown.

NUTRITION INFORMATION
SERVING SIZE: 1 serving   **CALORIES:** 157   **PROTEIN:** 11 g   **CARBS:** 18 g   **FAT:** 2 g

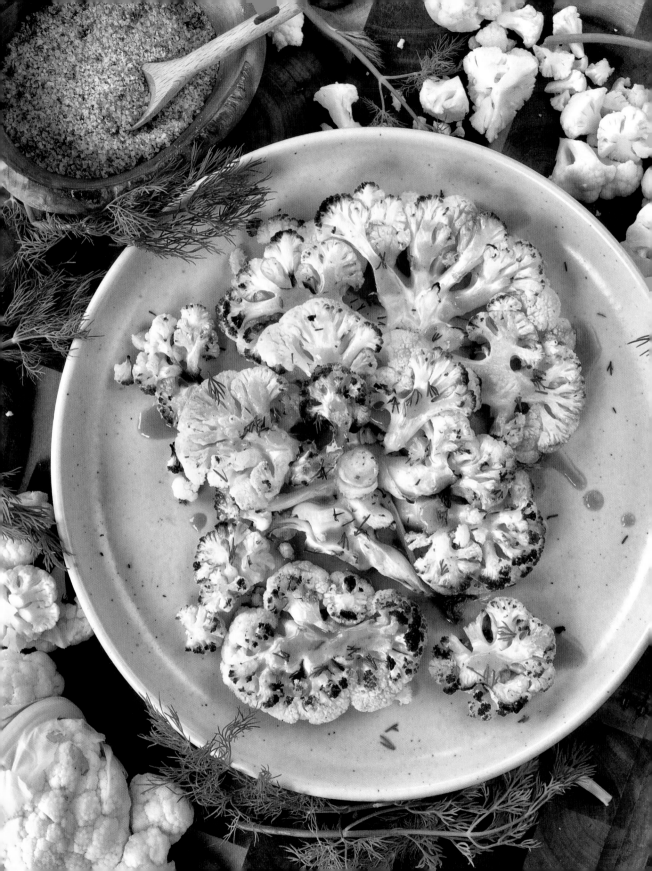

Roasted Cauliflower Steaks with Maple Mustard and Dill

SERVES 1 or 2

My Maple Mustard Dressing is versatile and really goes well with roasted cauliflower. I'll say it over and over: The keys to well-roasted cauliflower are to season it well with garlic salt, give it a light spray of oil, and roast it long enough to brown.

1 medium head cauliflower, sliced through the stem end into ½-inch-thick steaks

¼ teaspoon garlic salt, plus more if you like things garlicky

2 tablespoons Maple Mustard Dill Dressing (page 184)

1. Preheat the oven to 425°F. Line a baking sheet with parchment paper.

2. Arrange the cauliflower steaks in a single layer on the prepared baking sheet. Sprinkle each steak on both sides with the garlic salt. Roast for 20 to 30 minutes, or until just starting to brown. Dress with the maple mustard dressing and enjoy.

NOTE: You could also cut the cauliflower into florets and prepare them the same way as the steaks.

NUTRITION INFORMATION
SERVING SIZE: 1 serving   CALORIES: 107   PROTEIN: 6 g   CARBS: 16 g   FAT: 1 g

Green Beans with Sweet Soy Ginger Sauce

SERVES 1 OR 2

The secret to making these green beans even more delicious is letting them sit overnight in the soy ginger sauce. They soak up all the flavors of the sauce and make an amazing cold or heated dish the next day!

1 pound fresh or frozen green beans
¼ cup Sweet Soy Ginger Sauce (page 185)
¼ teaspoon sesame seeds, for garnish
¼ teaspoon chili flakes (optional)

1. Fill a large pot with a fitted lid with 2 inches of water and bring to a simmer over medium-high heat. Put the green beans in a steamer basket and place the basket in the pot. Cover and steam until the green beans are bright green and tender but not soft, 5 to 8 minutes.

2. Transfer the green beans to a medium bowl, add the sweet soy ginger sauce, and toss. Sprinkle with the sesame seeds and chili flakes, if desired. Serve immediately or let cool and store in the refrigerator in a lidded container to enjoy the next day.

NUTRITION INFORMATION
SERVING SIZE: 1 serving   **CALORIES:** 171   **PROTEIN:** 8 g   **CARBS:** 23 g   **FAT:** 1 g

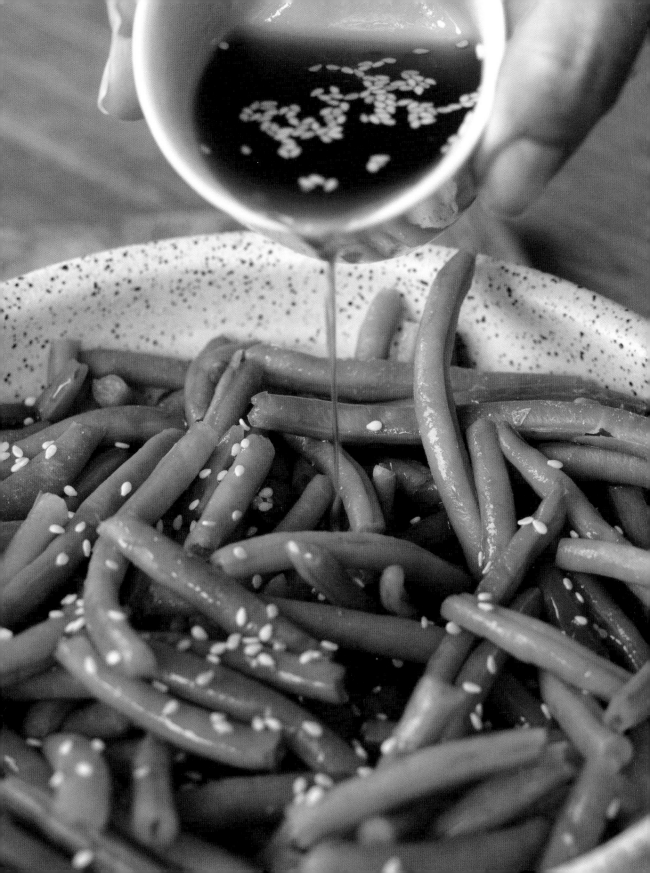

Bok Choy with Sweet Soy Ginger Sauce

The best bok choy is baby bok choy—at least, that's what my family is obsessed with. We grow it in our garden, and when it's steamed, dressed with my Sweet Soy Ginger Sauce, and garnished with sesame seeds, it's a fam favorite.

---

1 pound baby bok choy, ends trimmed, halved lengthwise

¼ cup Sweet Soy Ginger Sauce (page 185), or 3 tablespoons coconut aminos teriyaki sauce (I like Coconut Secret)

¼ teaspoon sesame seeds, for garnish

---

1. Fill a large pot with a fitted lid with 2 inches of water and bring to a simmer over medium-high heat. Put the bok choy in a steamer basket and place the basket in the pot. Cover and steam for 3 to 5 minutes, until the bok choy is fork-tender.

2. Transfer the bok choy to a medium bowl. Toss with the sweet soy ginger sauce or coconut aminos and sprinkle with the sesame seeds. Serve.

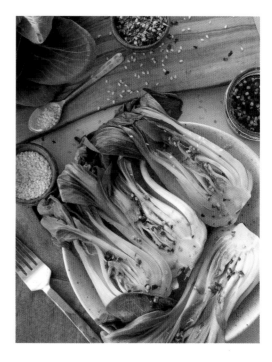

NUTRITION INFORMATION
SERVING SIZE: 1 serving   **CALORIES:** 103   **PROTEIN:** 8 g   **CARBS:** 13 g   **FAT:** 1 g

Caesar Dressing

If you miss having Caesar salad on a plant-based diet, then this dressing is for you! It is simple to put together and so delicious! If you like the flavor a little sharper, just add more caper brine and lemon juice.

NOTE: A thicker plant-based milk is what makes this dressing thick and creamy. My favorites are Westsoy soy milk and Three Trees Organics almond milk. If you can't find either of those or another thicker milk, use your favorite plain, unsweetened plant-based milk and add an extra ¼ cup cashews to thicken (this will only change the calories per tablespoon by about 5 calories). If you want an even thicker dressing, use less milk.

1 cup plain, unsweetened plant-based milk (see Note)

½ cup raw unsalted cashews

2 tablespoons fresh lemon juice

1 tablespoon whole-grain mustard or Dijon mustard

1 teaspoon capers in brine, plus 2 teaspoons of their brine

¾ teaspoon sea salt, plus more as needed

½ teaspoon garlic powder or minced fresh garlic

¼ teaspoon onion powder

⅛ teaspoon vegan Worcestershire sauce (I like Annie's)

⅛ teaspoon freshly ground black pepper, plus more as needed

1. In a blender, combine the milk, cashews, lemon juice, mustard, capers, caper brine, salt, garlic powder, onion powder, and Worcestershire sauce. Blend until smooth and creamy. Mix in the pepper, taste, and adjust the seasonings if needed.

2. Store in an airtight container in the refrigerator for up to 5 days.

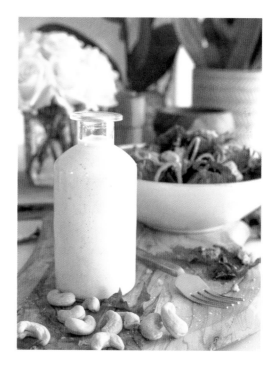

NUTRITION INFORMATION
SERVING SIZE: 1 tablespoon **CALORIES:** 22 **PROTEIN:** 1 g **CARBS:** 1 g **FAT:** 1.5 g

Cheeseless Cheese Sauce

MAKES ABOUT 4½ CUPS

Cheese sauce was the very first thing I set out to conquer as a new plant-based eater. I was a cheese addict, and I knew that if I was going to be successful on a plant-based diet, a delicious cheese sauce was going to be important. The nutritional yeast gives this sauce an extra cheesy flavor, not to mention B vitamins, but if you have an aversion to it, you can simply leave it out. I make this sauce every Sunday so we have it on hand to use throughout the week. It's perfect to pour over broccoli or to top a baked potato, but I use it for everything!

3 cups diced peeled white potatoes (see Note)

½ cup diced carrots (see Note)

½ cup raw unsalted cashews

3 tablespoons nutritional yeast (optional)

2 teaspoons garlic powder or minced fresh garlic

2 teaspoons sea salt

1¼ teaspoons fresh lemon juice

1 teaspoon onion powder

1. In a medium pot, combine the potatoes and carrots and add enough cold water to just cover them. Bring the water to a boil, then reduce the heat to maintain a simmer and cook until the potatoes and carrots are soft, 15 to 20 minutes. Drain the potatoes and carrots in a colander set over a bowl, then transfer to a high-speed blender; reserve the cooking water.

2. Add the cashews, nutritional yeast (if using), garlic powder, salt, lemon juice, and onion powder to the blender, along with 2 cups of the reserved cooking water. Blend until smooth, adding more of the reserved cooking water if you'd like a thinner consistency.

3. Let cool, then store in an airtight container in the refrigerator for up to 1 week.

NUT-FREE VARIATION: Replace the cashews with white beans or hemp hearts. Add just 1 cup of the reserved cooking water to start, then add more if you'd like a thinner sauce.

FAT-FREE VARIATION: Omit the cashews. Add just 1 cup of the reserved cooking water to start, then add more if you'd like a thinner consistency.

NUTRITION INFORMATION
SERVING SIZE: ¼ cup   CALORIES: 57   PROTEIN: 2 g   CARBS: 8 g   FAT: 2 g
SERVING SIZE: ¼ cup (nut-free, made with hemp hearts)   CALORIES: 49   PROTEIN: 2 g   CARBS: 8 g   FAT: 1 g
SERVING SIZE: ¼ cup (fat-free, made without cashews)   CALORIES: 55   PROTEIN: 1 g   CARBS: 7g   FAT: 0 g

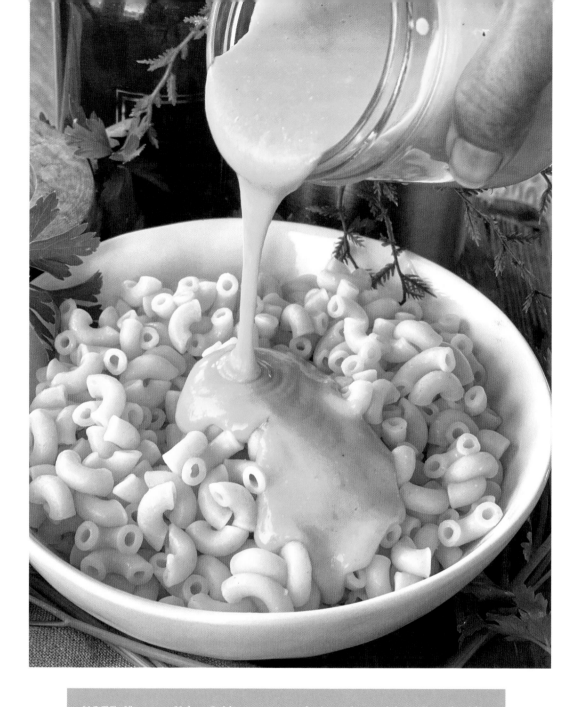

NOTE: If you use Yukon Gold potatoes, you don't need to peel them. To make this a white cheese sauce, omit the carrots. Also, this recipe calls for a high-speed blender, which will help you get the creamiest texture possible. If you have a less powerful blender, either grind the nuts or boil them whole for 7 minutes before blending, which will make them easier to break down.

BBQ Ranch

BBQ sauce is a very personal thing. Depending on who you are and where you're from and whether you like Texas or Kentucky or St. Louis–style barbecue, you might have strong feelings about your sauces. Regardless of your preference, I have the sauce for you: a ranch that gets its flavor from your favorite bottle of BBQ sauce. The base is cashews and soy milk, but the flavoring comes from whatever you like best for a creamy, smoky dressing! It's also delicious over sandwiches and wraps, and it's great for dipping oven-baked fries in.

1 cup plain, unsweetened plant-based milk (see Note on page 175)

½ cup raw unsalted cashews (see Note)

¼ cup plus 2 tablespoons BBQ sauce of your choice

2 tablespoons distilled white vinegar

¾ teaspoon sea salt, plus more as needed

½ teaspoon garlic powder or minced fresh garlic

¼ teaspoon onion powder

1. In a blender, combine the milk, cashews, BBQ sauce, vinegar, salt, garlic powder, and onion powder. Blend until smooth and creamy.

2. Taste and adjust the seasoning with more salt, if needed. Store the sauce in an airtight container in the refrigerator for up to 5 days.

NUTRITION INFORMATION
SERVING SIZE: 1 tablespoon   **CALORIES:** 26   **PROTEIN:** 1 g   **CARBS:** 3 g   **FAT:** 1 g
SERVING SIZE: 1 tablespoon (nut-free, made with hemp hearts)   **CALORIES:** 22   **PROTEIN:** 1 g   **CARBS:** 1.8 g   **FAT:** 1.2 g

Southwest Ranch

I love ranch dressing in all its forms. This one is simple and tasty. If you want more heat, try adding your favorite hot sauce to the mix!

**1 cup plain, unsweetened plant-based milk
(see Note on page 175)**

½ cup raw unsalted cashews (see Note on page 175)

2 tablespoons distilled white vinegar

2½ teaspoons chili powder

¾ teaspoon sea salt, plus more if needed

½ teaspoon garlic powder or minced fresh garlic

¼ teaspoon onion powder

Zest of 1 lime

**1 tablespoon chopped fresh
cilantro leaves (optional)**

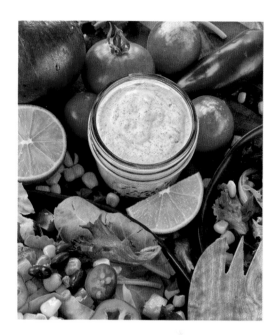

1. In a blender, combine the milk, cashews, vinegar, chili powder, salt, garlic powder, onion powder, and lime zest. Blend until smooth and creamy.

2. Transfer the dressing to a lidded container and mix in the cilantro, if desired. Taste and adjust the seasoning with more salt, if needed. Store in the refrigerator for up to 5 days.

NUTRITION INFORMATION
SERVING SIZE: 1 tablespoon **CALORIES:** 19 **PROTEIN:** 1 g **CARBS:** 1 g **FAT:** 1 g
SERVING SIZE: 1 tablespoon (nut-free, made with hemp hearts) **CALORIES:** 19 **PROTEIN:** 1.2 g **CARBS:** 0.2 g **FAT:** 1.3 g

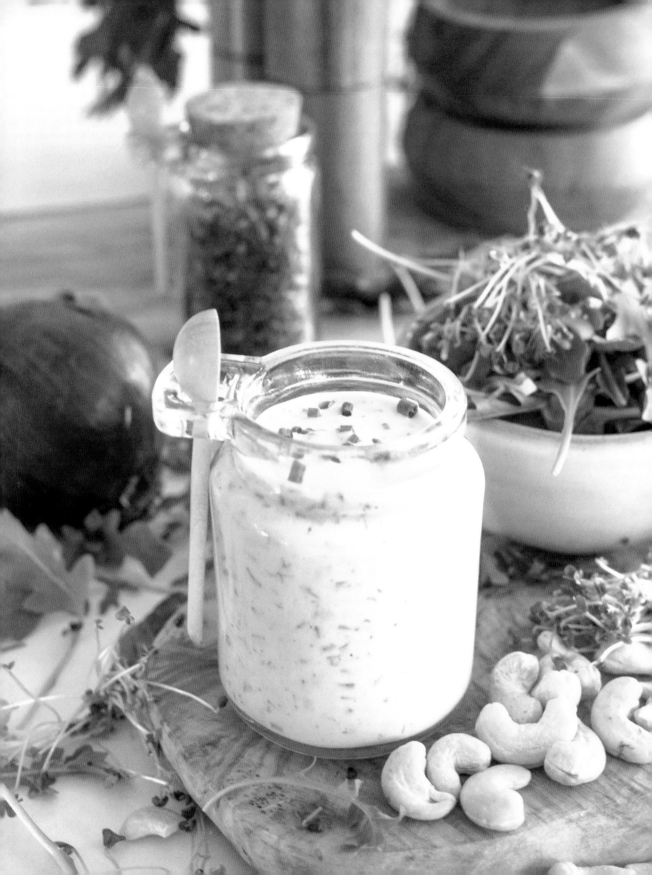

Cashew Ranch Dressing

MAKES
1½
CUPS

If you're not a lover of salads, like I used to be, then try this ranch. For me, salad is synonymous with ranch dressing, but for my first six months of plant-based eating, I couldn't find a ranch without a lot of fat and calories. Consequently, I didn't enjoy many salads, and it took me months of playing with this recipe to finally get it to be the ranch I was looking for. The key, I learned, is the thickness of the plant milk you choose. I use Westsoy soy milk or Three Trees Organics almond milk for this because they lend the best flavor and creaminess.

1. In a blender, combine the milk, cashews, vinegar, salt, garlic powder, onion powder, and a pinch of pepper. Blend until smooth and creamy.

2. Transfer the dressing to a lidded container and mix in the parsley and dill (if using). Taste and adjust the seasoning with more salt and pepper, if needed. Store in the refrigerator for up to 5 days.

**1 cup plain, unsweetened plant-based milk
(see Note on page 175)**
½ cup raw unsalted cashews (see Note on page 175)
2 tablespoons distilled white vinegar
¾ teaspoon sea salt, plus more if needed
½ teaspoon garlic powder or minced fresh garlic
¼ teaspoon onion powder
Freshly ground black pepper
1 teaspoon dried parsley
Pinch of dried dill (optional)

NUTRITION INFORMATION
SERVING SIZE: 1 tablespoon   **CALORIES:** 18   **PROTEIN:** 1 g   **CARBS:** 1 g   **FAT:** 1 g
SERVING SIZE: 1 tablespoon (nut-free, made with hemp hearts)   **CALORIES:** 19   **PROTEIN:** 1.2 g   **CARBS:** 0.2 g   **FAT:** 1.3 g

Thousand Island

This dressing is my go-to not only for salad but also as a dip and even as a sandwich or wrap spread. I especially love dipping onion rings in it!

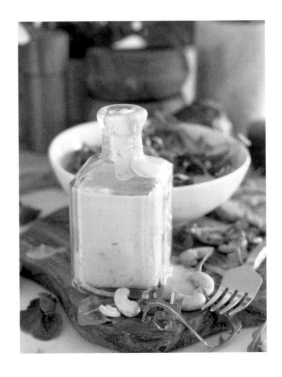

1 cup plain, unsweetened plant-based milk (see Note on page 175)

½ cup raw unsalted cashews (see Note on page 175)

¼ cup plus 1 tablespoon ketchup

3 tablespoons sweet relish

2 tablespoons distilled white vinegar

¾ teaspoon sea salt

½ teaspoon garlic powder or minced fresh garlic

¼ teaspoon onion powder

In a blender, combine the milk, cashews, ketchup, relish, vinegar, salt, garlic powder, and onion powder. Blend until smooth and creamy. Store in an airtight container in the refrigerator for 3 to 5 days.

NUTRITION INFORMATION
SERVING SIZE: 1 tablespoon   **CALORIES:** 23   **PROTEIN:** 1 g   **CARBS:** 2 g   **FAT:** 1 g

Thai Peanut Sauce

MAKES
5
TABLESPOONS

If you love peanut sauce, you'll love this recipe. I switched out the peanut butter for lower-fat, lower-calorie powdered peanut butter and then added just a few more ingredients. If you want to reduce the calories even more, try sweetening the dressing with stevia drops instead of the maple syrup. You can also add ⅛ teaspoon toasted sesame oil for extra flavor—that only adds 5 calories and ½ gram of fat to the entire recipe!

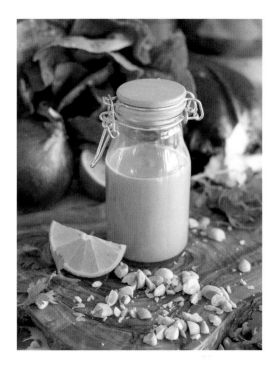

½ cup powdered peanut butter (I like PB2)

2 tablespoons pure maple syrup, or 4 drops stevia

1 tablespoon fresh lime juice

1 tablespoon low-sodium soy sauce

½ teaspoon oil-free chili paste
(I like sambal oelek; optional)

⅛ teaspoon ground ginger

⅛ teaspoon toasted sesame oil (optional)

In a medium bowl, combine the powdered peanut butter, maple syrup, lime juice, soy sauce, chili paste (if using), ginger, and sesame oil (if using). Add 3 tablespoons water and whisk well to combine. Store in an airtight container in the refrigerator for up to 4 days.

NUTRITION INFORMATION
SERVING SIZE: 2 tablespoons   CALORIES: 70   PROTEIN: 6 g   CARBS: 8 g   FAT: 1 g

Maple Mustard Dressing, Three Ways

This is hands down one of the easiest dressings you can make, and takes literally two minutes, maybe. You can play with different flavors and add this to your salads and roasted vegetable dishes.

In a jar with a tight lid, combine all the ingredients and shake vigorously. Store in an airtight container in the refrigerator for up to 1 week.

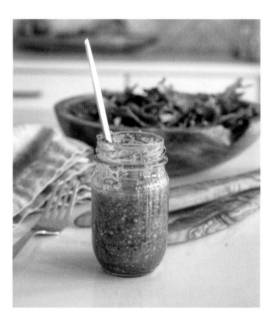

BASIC VERSION:
¼ cup Dijon mustard
¼ cup pure maple syrup

SMOKY MAPLE MUSTARD DRESSING:
¼ cup Dijon mustard
¼ cup pure maple syrup
¼ teaspoon smoked paprika

DILL MAPLE MUSTARD DRESSING:
¼ cup Dijon mustard
¼ cup pure maple syrup
Pinch of dried dill

NUTRITION INFORMATION
SERVING SIZE: 2 tablespoons   **CALORIES:** 67   **PROTEIN:** 1 g   **CARBS:** 14 g   **FAT:** 1 g

Sweet Soy Ginger Sauce

My husband and I love going to Young's Cafe, a family-owned Vietnamese restaurant in our town. We've been eating there for about twenty years, and the owner treats us like family. The chef makes the most delicious ginger sauce, and I always order it to have with my steamed rice and veggies. This is my take on that dressing. I love to soak my steamed green beans in this dressing overnight and eat them the next day after they've absorbed all the delicious flavors.

to combine. Store in an airtight container in the refrigerator for up to 1 week.

NOTE: The toasted sesame oil is optional; it adds just 10 calories and ½ gram of fat to the entire recipe.

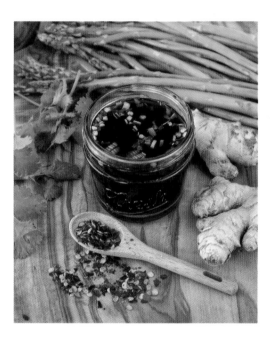

¼ **cup low-sodium soy sauce**

¼ **cup rice vinegar**

2 tablespoons pure maple syrup

½ **teaspoon grated fresh ginger, or ⅛ teaspoon ground ginger**

½ **teaspoon minced garlic, or ⅛ teaspoon garlic powder**

¼ **teaspoon toasted sesame oil (optional; see Note)**

In a medium bowl, whisk together the soy sauce, vinegar, maple syrup, ginger, garlic, and sesame oil (if using). Add ½ cup water and whisk

NUTRITION INFORMATION
SERVING SIZE: ¼ cup   **CALORIES:** 39   **PROTEIN:** 1 g   **CARBS:** 8 g   **FAT:** 0 g

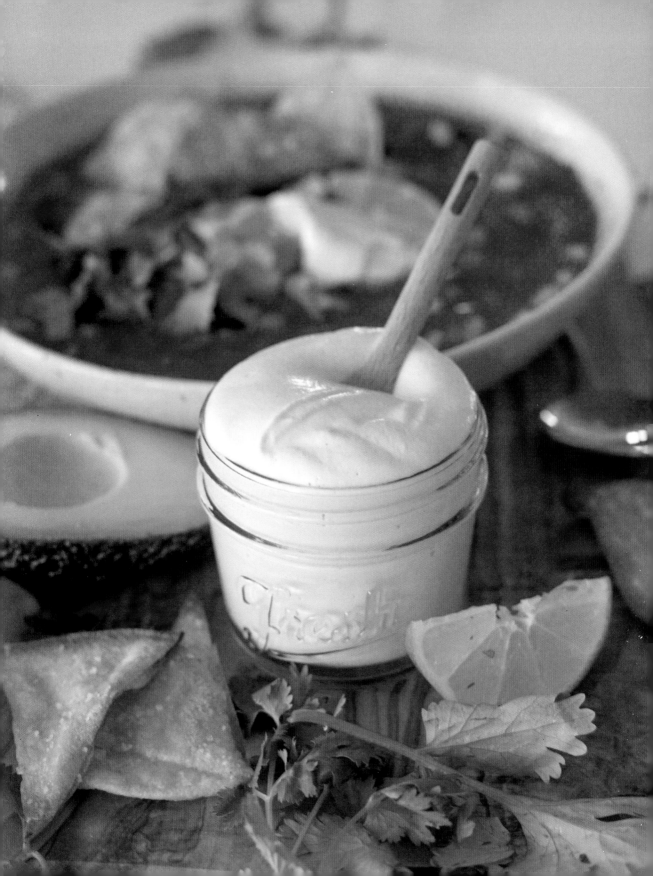

Cashew Sour Cream

What is it about sour cream that adds so much happiness to a taco or burrito? All I know is that if loving sour cream is wrong, I don't want to be right. This simple vegan sour cream comes together so easily and dresses up burrito bowls and tortilla soup so well that you won't even think about full-fat dairy sour cream.

1 cup raw, unsalted cashews, soaked overnight (see Note)

¼ cup fresh lemon juice

2 teaspoons distilled white vinegar

½ teaspoon sea salt

2 drops stevia, or ¼ teaspoon pure maple syrup

Drain and rinse the cashews. Transfer them to a blender and add the lemon juice, vinegar, salt, stevia, and ½ cup water. Blend until smooth. Store in an airtight container in the refrigerator for up to 5 days.

NOTE: If you forget to soak your cashews overnight, just put them in a bowl, pour boiling water over them, and let them soak for 4 hours. They'll soften enough for this to whip up quickly.

NUTRITION INFORMATION
SERVING SIZE: 1 tablespoon CALORIES: 31 PROTEIN: 1 g CARBS: 2 g FAT: 2 g

Pickled Onions

MAKES

2

CUPS

I know pickling sounds labor-intensive and complicated, but I'm telling you, these pickled onions are easy, absolutely delicious, and add so much flavor. In the part of the Yucatán where I'm from, hardly a dish is served without them. They always accompany beans and rice.

1 large red onion, thinly sliced
1 cup distilled white vinegar
Pinch of sea salt
Pinch of dried oregano

1. Place the onion in a quart-size heatproof glass jar. Set aside.

2. In a small nonreactive pot, combine the vinegar, salt, oregano, and 1 cup water. Bring to a boil over medium heat, then remove the pot from the heat.

3. Pour the mixture over the onions and let cool completely. Seal the jar and store in the refrigerator. They're ready to enjoy as soon as they're cool, and will keep for 1 to 2 weeks.

NUTRITION INFORMATION
SERVING SIZE: ¼ cup **CALORIES:** 8 **PROTEIN:** 0 g **CARBS:** 1 g **FAT:** 0.0 g

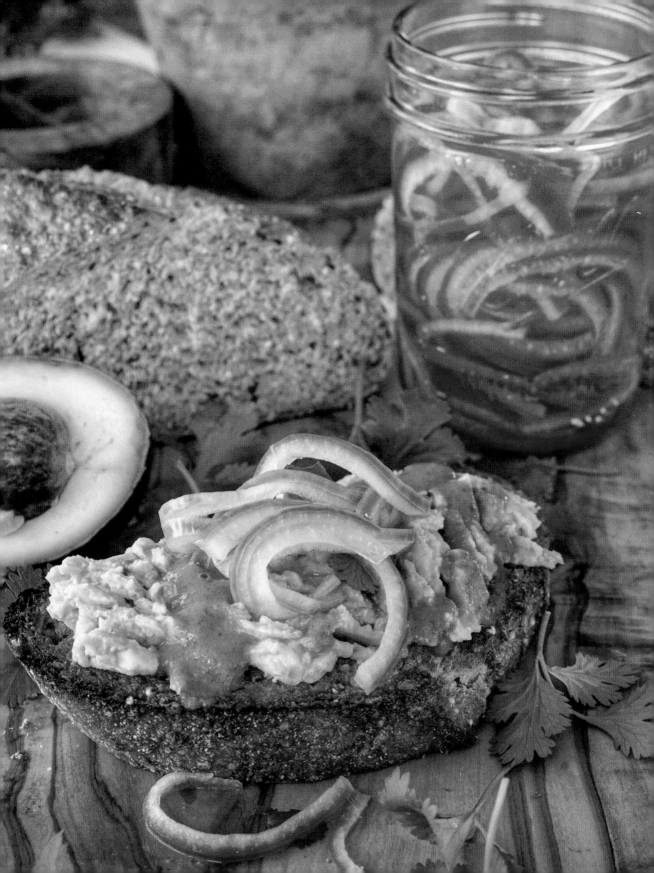

Mushroom Gravy

Coming up with a low-fat gravy that still feels creamy and satisfying was definitely a challenge. But after much trial and error, I made this mushroom gravy, and it's an absolute delight! The key is a good, creamy plant-based milk—I personally love the almond milk by Three Trees Organics or the plain, unsweetened soy milk by WestSoy, which has about 100 calories per cup. If you can't find those particular milks, look for a plain, unsweetened plant-based milk with a similar calorie count (or use one with fewer calories if you prefer, of course!).

16 ounces white mushrooms or baby bella (cremini) mushrooms, chopped

¼ teaspoon sea salt, plus more as needed

2 cups plain, unsweetened plant-based milk

1 teaspoon fresh lemon juice

½ teaspoon poultry seasoning

¼ teaspoon garlic powder, plus more as needed

¼ teaspoon onion powder, plus more as needed

Freshly ground black pepper

1. In a large nonstick sauté pan, combine the mushrooms with a splash of water and season with the salt. Cook over medium-high heat, stirring occasionally, until the mushrooms are soft, 8 to 10 minutes.

2. Transfer the mushrooms to a blender and add the milk, lemon juice, poultry seasoning, garlic powder, onion powder, and a pinch each of salt and pepper. Blend until smooth. Taste and adjust the seasoning, if needed.

3. Let cool completely, then store in an airtight container in the refrigerator for up to 3 days.

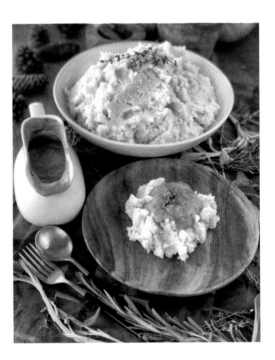

NUTRITION INFORMATION

SERVING SIZE: ½ cup   CALORIES: 48   PROTEIN: 3 g   CARBS: 2 g   FAT: 3 g

Raspberry-Lime Sauce

If it takes a minute or less to make, I'm all about it! This is simple, but holy moly, it's so good on dishes that include beans and sweet potatoes! Try this on the Sweet Potato Tacos on page 115, and you'll be a major fan of this simple combination, too. Roasted sweet potato fries are excellent dipped into this as well; putting this sauce in a little dish on the side is how I got my kids to start enjoying sweet potato.

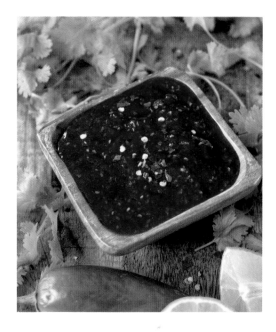

¼ cup raspberry jelly, sweetened with fruit juice
1½ teaspoons fresh lime juice
Pinch of chili flakes

In a medium bowl, whisk together the jelly, lime juice, chili flakes, and 1½ teaspoons water. Store in an airtight container in the refrigerator for up to 5 days.

NUTRITION INFORMATION
SERVING SIZE: 2 tablespoons   **CALORIES:** 91   **PROTEIN:** 0 g   **CARBS:** 23 g   **FAT:** 0.0 g

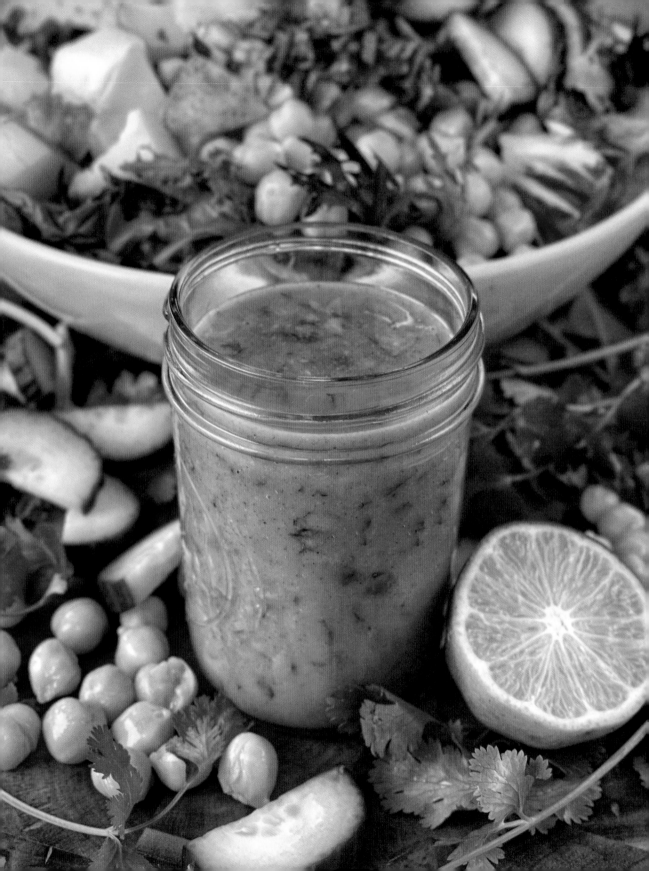

Cilantro-Curry Dressing

MAKES
1/2
CUP

A nice change from the usual creamy dressings, this cilantro dressing has incredible flavor balanced by the kick of the mustard and curry and the sweetness of the maple syrup. It's a great addition to a chickpea and cucumber salad. You can save even more calories if you use an all-natural sugar-free maple syrup sweetened with stevia or monk fruit.

In a small airtight container, combine the Dijon, maple syrup, cilantro, lime juice, and curry powder. Cover with the lid and give the container a good shake. Store the dressing in the refrigerator for up to 1 week.

NOTE: Feel free to adjust the amount of curry to suit your taste.

¼ cup Dijon mustard
¼ cup pure maple syrup
1 tablespoon chopped fresh cilantro leaves
2 teaspoons fresh lime juice
½ teaspoon yellow curry powder (see Note)

NUTRITION INFORMATION
SERVING SIZE: 2 tablespoons **CALORIES:** 68 **PROTEIN:** 1 g **CARBS:** 14 g **FAT:** 1 g

CHAPTER 4

Snacks and Cravings

Cilantro-Curry Hummus

MAKES ABOUT
1
CUP

I don't know why it took me so long to think about adding curry powder to my hummus, but once I did . . . wow! I then discovered that adding cilantro and lime juice makes all the flavors work together for a hummus that really pops. This is my go-to hummus, and I use it as a spread for sandwiches as well as a wonderful snack with fresh-cut vegetables.

1 (15-ounce) can cannellini beans or white beans of your choice, drained and rinsed

2 tablespoons fresh lime juice

1 tablespoon fresh lemon juice

½ to 1 teaspoon curry powder, depending on how strong you want the flavor

¼ teaspoon ground turmeric

¼ teaspoon sea salt, plus more as needed

2 tablespoons finely chopped fresh cilantro (see Note)

1. In a food processor or high-speed blender, combine the beans, lime juice, lemon juice, curry powder, turmeric, and salt. Process until smooth. Taste and adjust the seasoning with more salt, if desired, and fold in the cilantro. Serve with fresh vegetables or as a sandwich spread.

2. Store leftovers in an airtight container in the refrigerator for up to 7 days.

> **NOTE:** If you don't like the taste of cilantro or don't have it on hand, feel free to use parsley instead.

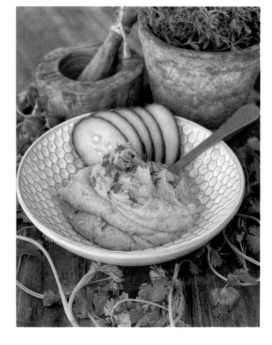

NUTRITION INFORMATION
SERVING SIZE: ¼ cup **CALORIES:** 72 **PROTEIN:** 5 g **CARBS:** 7 g **FAT:** 0 g

Smoky Tomato Hummus

MAKES ABOUT
1
CUP

I'm always thinking of new ways to make over a hummus recipe because that translates to a new dip or spread I can add to wraps and sandwiches. This hummus makes an excellent spread for a vegetable-filled sandwich and is also excellent with fresh-cut vegetables as a dip. It has a deep smoky flavor that adds heartiness to your meal.

1 (15-ounce) can chickpeas, drained and rinsed

½ cup sun-dried tomatoes, soaked for 10 minutes in hot water and drained

2 tablespoons fresh orange juice

2 tablespoons fresh lemon juice

1 tablespoon Dijon mustard

1 teaspoon smoked paprika

½ teaspoon garlic powder or minced fresh garlic

½ teaspoon sea salt

½ teaspoon liquid smoke (optional)

¼ teaspoon onion powder

1. In a food processor or high-speed blender, combine the chickpeas, sun-dried tomatoes, orange juice, lemon juice, Dijon, paprika, garlic powder, salt, liquid smoke (if using), and onion powder. Process until smooth and serve with fresh vegetables as a dip or as a sandwich spread.

2. Store leftovers in an airtight container in the refrigerator for up to 7 days.

NUTRITION INFORMATION
SERVING SIZE: ¼ cup   **CALORIES:** 131   **PROTEIN:** 6 g   **CARBS:** 18 g   **FAT:** 2 g

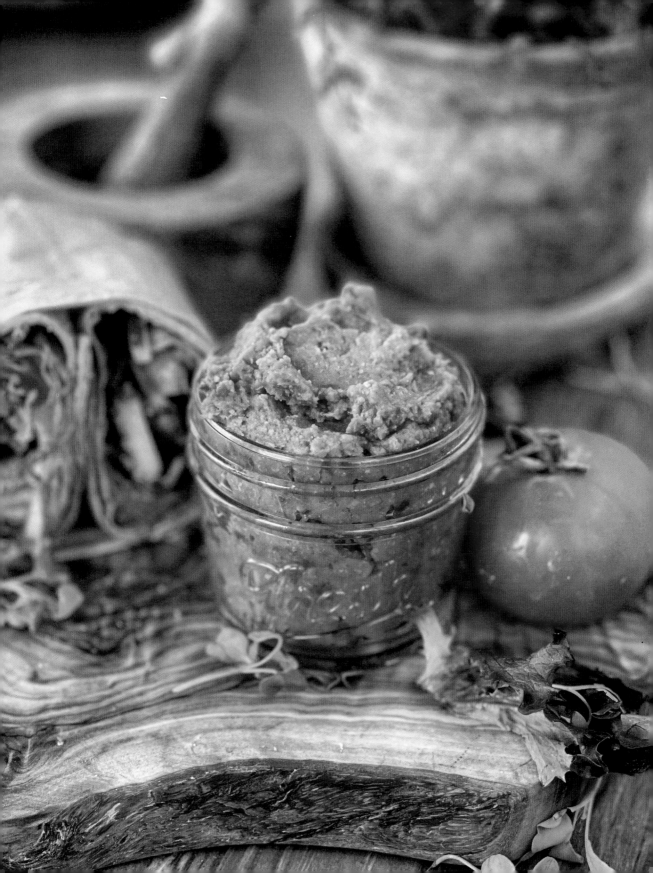

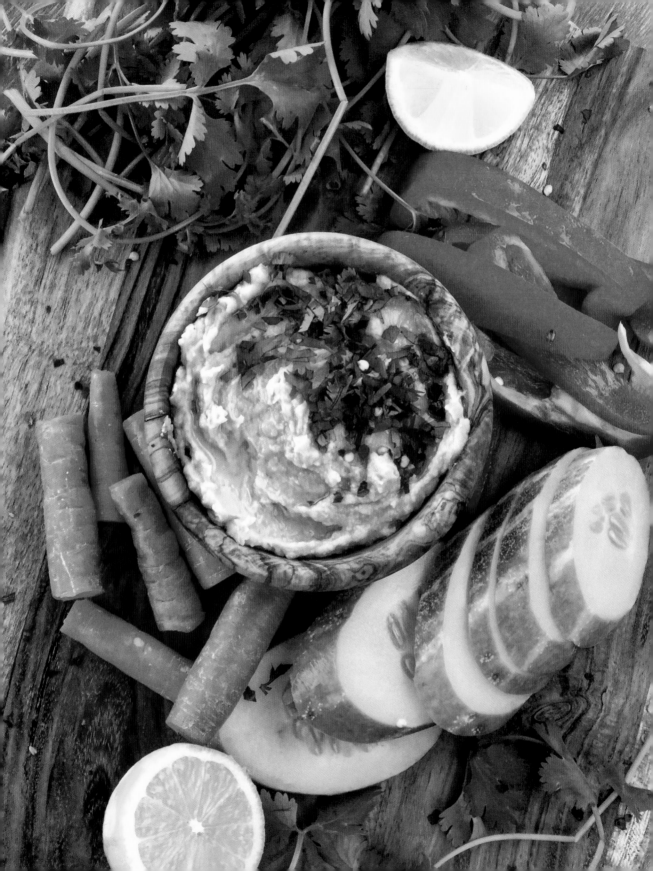

Creamy Cannellini Hummus

MAKES ABOUT 1 CUP

I love a creamy hummus, which is usually achieved with a lot of oil or tahini—or both. Those ingredients make a delicious hummus but also a heavy one, high in fat and calories. Here I go for that richness by swapping out chickpeas for cannellini beans, which are creamy and buttery and fill in for the oil and tahini to make this hummus a great spread or dip for fresh vegetables!

1 (15-ounce) can cannellini beans, drained and rinsed

1 tablespoon fresh lemon juice, plus more for serving

1 tablespoon low-sodium soy sauce

1 teaspoon Dijon mustard

1 teaspoon garlic powder or minced fresh garlic

⅛ teaspoon ground cumin (optional)

Sea salt

Chopped fresh cilantro leaves, for garnish

Chili flakes, for garnish

1. In a food processor or high-speed blender, combine the beans, lemon juice, soy sauce, Dijon, garlic powder, cumin (if using), and a pinch of salt. Process until smooth. Taste and adjust the seasoning with more salt, if needed.

2. Transfer the dip to a serving bowl and drizzle with lemon juice. Garnish with cilantro and chili flakes, then serve. Store leftovers in an airtight container in the refrigerator for up to 7 days.

NUTRITION INFORMATION
SERVING SIZE: ¼ cup   CALORIES: 75   PROTEIN: 5 g   CARBS: 7 g   FAT: 0 g

Easy Eggless Egg Salad

MAKES ABOUT
1
CUP

Egg salad was a staple in my house growing up. Believe it or not, my mom would often make it for breakfast. She would warm it up and serve it to us on toast, and it was somehow always so comforting. I have passed that tradition on to my children, but my version of the salad uses protein-rich chickpeas, which works for our plant-based lifestyle. This also makes an excellent spread for lunches and a great dip to serve with rice crackers and veggies when you have company.

1 (15-ounce) can chickpeas, drained and rinsed
3 tablespoons Cashew Ranch Dressing (page 181)
2 tablespoons yellow mustard
¼ teaspoon sea salt, plus more as needed
Freshly ground black pepper

1. In a medium bowl, use a fork, potato masher, or your hands to mash the chickpeas, leaving them somewhat chunky. Add the ranch, mustard, salt, and a pinch of pepper. Mix well. Taste and adjust the seasoning with more salt and pepper, if needed. Serve with fresh vegetables as a dip, on salad greens, or as a sandwich spread.

2. Store leftovers in an airtight container in the refrigerator for up to 5 days.

NUTRITION INFORMATION
SERVING SIZE: ¼ cup   **CALORIES:** 104 g   **PROTEIN:** 5 g   **CARBS:** 11 g   **FAT:** 3 g

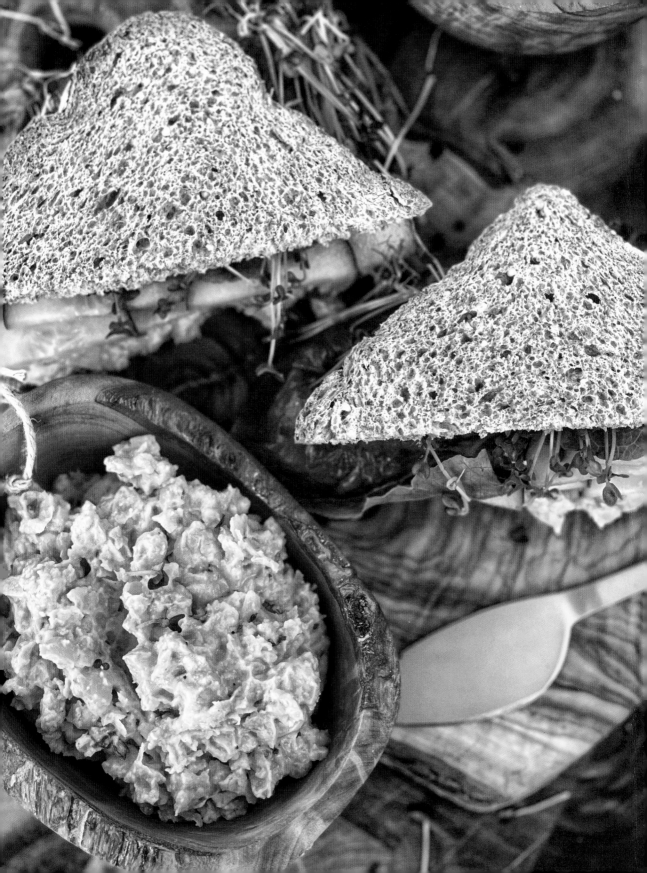

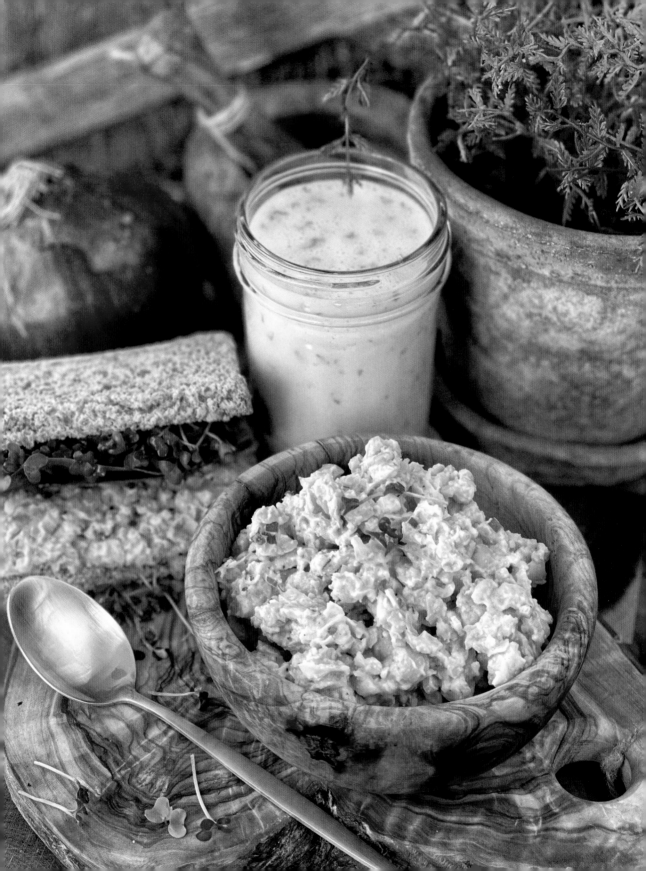

Chickpea "Chicken" Salad

MAKES ABOUT 1 CUP

This is one of my favorite recipes because it's so versatile. It's crunchy and flavorful, and packed full of nutrition, too. I love to bring this to a barbecue to serve as a dip with crackers and vegetables or scooped over greens. It also makes a delicious filling for a sandwich or wrap that you can take with you to work or on a picnic!

1 (15-ounce) can chickpeas, drained and rinsed

2 tablespoons minced red onion

2 tablespoons minced celery

¼ cup plus 1 tablespoon Cashew Ranch Dressing (page 181)

Sea salt and freshly ground black pepper

1. In a medium bowl, use a fork, potato masher, or your hands to mash the chickpeas, leaving them somewhat chunky but no whole chickpeas remaining. Add the onion, celery, and ranch and mix well. Taste and season with salt and pepper. Serve with fresh cut vegetables, over salad greens, or as a sandwich spread.

2. Store leftovers in an airtight container in the refrigerator for up to 5 days.

NUTRITION INFORMATION
SERVING SIZE: ¼ cup   **CALORIES:** 121   **PROTEIN:** 6 g   **CARBS:** 12 g   **FAT:** 4 g

Roasted Chickpeas, Two Ways

MAKES ABOUT
1
CUP

I used to have a major potato chip habit that I was in need of breaking. I just love something crunchy and salty! Then along came roasted chickpeas to save the day. These are quick and easy to make, and every bit as satisfying as a bag of chips! Don't be afraid to give the chickpeas a light spray of avocado oil to help them crisp up, which will add to your overall satisfaction. You'll be surprised how far a little oil can go in adding crispiness—you don't need tablespoons of oil to make these chickpeas crispy, so you won't be adding loads of fat and calories.

Smoky Roasted Chickpeas

1 (15-ounce) can chickpeas, drained and rinsed
¼ teaspoon garlic powder
¼ teaspoon smoked paprika
¼ teaspoon sea salt, plus more if needed
⅛ teaspoon onion powder
Avocado oil cooking spray

1. Preheat the oven or air fryer to 425°F. If roasting in the oven, line a rimmed baking sheet with parchment paper.

2. In a medium bowl, season the chickpeas with the garlic powder, paprika, salt, and onion powder. Toss to coat well.

3. Spread the chickpeas over the prepared baking sheet or in the basket of the air fryer and lightly spray with avocado oil. Cook for 10 to 13 minutes, until the chickpeas are golden and crispy. Taste and adjust the seasoning with more salt, if needed. Serve hot or at room temperature as a snack or salad topping.

4. Store leftovers in an airtight container at room temperature for up to 2 days.

NUTRITION INFORMATION
SERVING SIZE: ¼ cup   **CALORIES:** 57   **PROTEIN:** 3 g   **CARBS:** 7 g   **FAT:** 1 g

Curry-Roasted Chickpeas

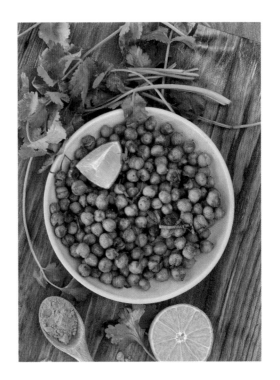

1 (15-ounce) can chickpeas, drained and rinsed

1½ teaspoons curry powder

½ teaspoon garlic powder

¼ teaspoon onion powder

¼ teaspoon sea salt, plus more as needed

Avocado oil cooking spray

1. Preheat the oven or air fryer to 425°F. If roasting in the oven, line a rimmed baking sheet with parchment paper.

2. In a medium bowl, season the chickpeas with the curry powder, garlic powder, onion powder, and salt. Toss to coat well.

3. Spread the chickpeas over the prepared baking sheet or in the basket of the air fryer and lightly spray with avocado oil. Cook for 10 to 13 minutes, until the chickpeas are golden and crispy. Taste and adjust the seasoning with more salt, if needed. Serve hot or at room temperature as a snack or salad topping.

4. Store leftovers in an airtight container at room temperature for up to 2 days.

NUTRITION INFORMATION
SERVING SIZE: ¼ cup   CALORIES: 54   PROTEIN: 3 g   CARBS: 7 g   FAT: 1 g

Weight Loss–Friendly Granola

MAKES
3½
CUPS

We make this granola every Sunday so we have it on hand for the week. We use it everywhere throughout the day: as a topping for fruit and yogurt and our homemade banana "nice creams." It's versatile and delicious, and the flavor combinations you can make are endless! But what makes this granola super special is that it's completely free of oil. Commercial granolas are loaded with fat and calories, but when you make granola at home, you decide what goes in it.

---

3 cups rolled oats
½ cup pure maple syrup
1 teaspoon pure vanilla extract
1 teaspoon pure almond extract

---

1. Preheat the oven to 375°F. Line a baking sheet with parchment paper.

2. In a medium bowl, combine the oats, maple syrup, vanilla, and almond extract. Mix well to combine.

3. Spread the mixture over the prepared baking sheet and bake for 10 minutes. Remove the baking sheet from the oven and carefully mix the granola. Return it to the oven and bake for 10 minutes more, or until the granola is golden brown.

4. Let the granola cool completely, then store in an airtight container at room temperature for up to 5 days.

NUTRITION INFORMATION
SERVING SIZE: ½ cup   **CALORIES:** 190   **PROTEIN:** 5 g   **CABS:** 35 g   **FAT:** 2 g

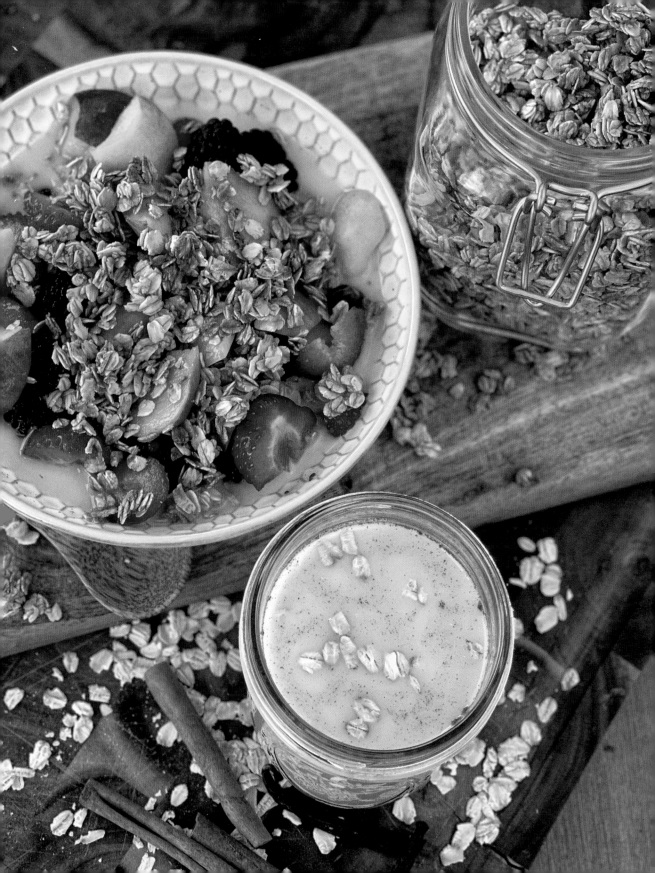

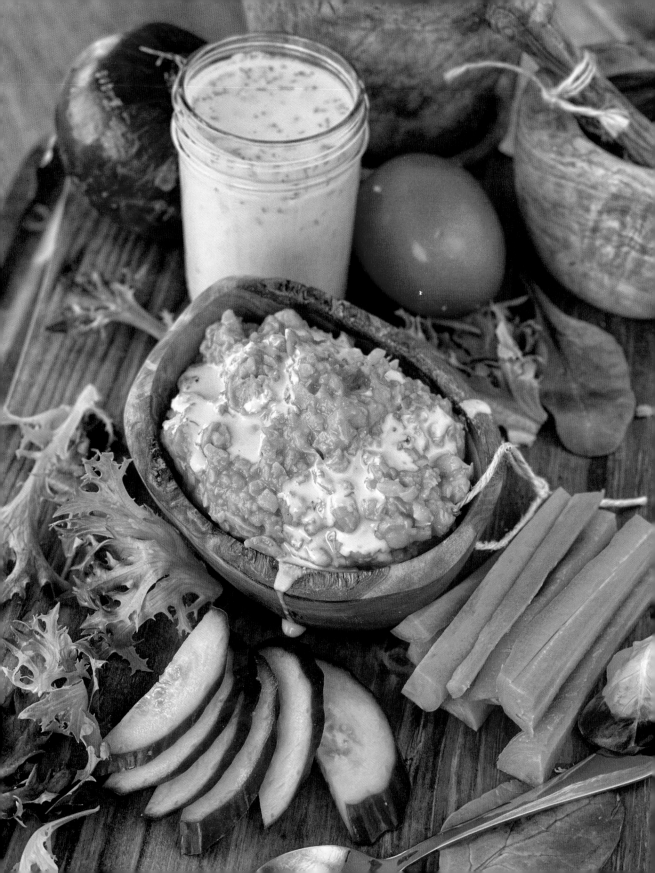

Buffalo Chickpea Dip

MAKES
1
CUP

My husband and I were invited to a friend's house for a Super Bowl party and were asked to bring a dip. Now, this was going to be a house full of mostly men, and men who loved meat. As a plant-based eater, I thought the best course of action would be to make a dip that tastes like Buffalo wings. That led me to topping this very simple preparation of mashed chickpeas drizzled with my Cashew Ranch Dressing and served with fresh-cut cucumbers and carrots. Instant hit! This would also be delicious as a filling for sandwiches and wraps, or scooped over greens as a salad.

1 (15-ounce) can chickpeas, drained and rinsed

3 tablespoons low-fat or fat-free wing sauce (I like Frank's RedHot in mild)

Southwest Ranch dressing (optional; page 179)

1. In a medium bowl, use a fork, potato masher, or your hands to mash the chickpeas, but leave some of their chunky texture. Add the wing sauce and mix well. Serve drizzled with optional ranch and cut cucumbers for dipping. This also makes a great spread for sandwiches and wraps, as well as a tasty salad topping.

2. Store leftovers in an airtight container in the refrigerator for up to 5 days.

NUTRITION INFORMATION
SERVING SIZE: ¼ cup   **CALORIES:** 97   **PROTEIN:** 4 g   **CARBS:** 11 g   **FAT:** 3 g

Baked Corn Tortilla Chips

SERVES
2

Oh, tortilla chips, how I love you. Chips and salsa, chips and guac, chips and bean dip, I love it all. The problem is, you don't love me—nor are you good for me. So I had to find a way to make this relationship work! Turns out, you can just cut up some corn tortillas, season them, and bake them, and you have yourself some low-fat, lower-calorie tortilla chips. (And if you give these a light spray of oil, no one will ever know they aren't fried!)

---

4 (6-inch) corn tortillas, cut into triangles

¼ teaspoon sea salt

½ cup salsa, store-bought or homemade (optional)

½ cup Cheese Sauce (page 176), warmed (optional)

---

1. Preheat the oven to 400°F. Spread the tortilla triangles over a baking sheet in a single layer, sprinkle with salt, and bake for 8 to 10 minutes, until just golden. Be sure to keep an eye on them—they burn quickly!

2. Serve with cheese sauce (page 176), Black Bean Salsa (page 213), or any of the chickpea dips.

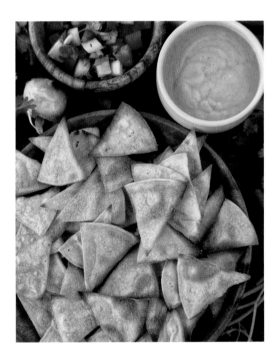

NUTRITION INFORMATION
SERVING SIZE: 1 serving with ¼ cup salsa and ¼ cup Cheese Sauce   **CALORIES:** 180   **PROTEIN:** 5 g   **CARBS:** 30 g   **FAT:** 3 g

Microwave Potato Chips

SERVES

2

I love potatoes in all their various forms, but potato chips take the cake! These are easy to make in the microwave, and you can flavor them any way you want. If you like salt-and-vinegar chips, try lightly spraying these with vinegar and seasoning them with salt before you microwave them.

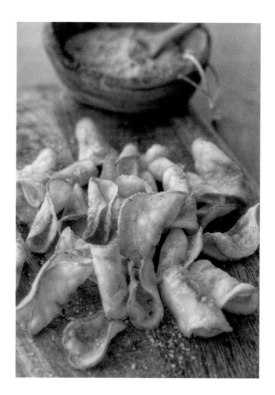

2 medium Yukon Gold potatoes
Garlic salt

1. Using a mandoline or sharp knife, cut the pota-toes into very thin slices.

2. Arrange the slices in a microwave potato chip maker, or line a dinner plate with parchment paper and place the slices in a single layer.

3. Sprinkle with the garlic salt and microwave on high for about 5 minutes, until they are crispy and lightly browned. Allow chips to cool com-pletely before serving.

NUTRITION INFORMATION
SERVING SIZE: 1 serving   **CALORIES:** 138   **PROTEIN:** 3 g   **CARBS:** 27 g   **FAT:** 0.2 g

Truffle Garlic Popcorn

SERVES
2

If you've never used truffle salt before, you're going to thank me! It has tons of rich, savory flavor that's super satisfying and enjoyable. Popcorn is one of those foods that's just plain fun to eat, but it's crazy how fattening it can be when you start cooking and seasoning it with oil and butter! Air-popping popcorn will save lots of calories, and by adding flavor-packed seasonings, you won't miss the fat. You can get those seasonings to stick by spraying the popcorn very lightly with water or oil. You'll get all the flavor and fun of the popcorn without all the fat and calories—plus, it's a whole grain!

¼ cup plus 2 tablespoons unpopped popcorn kernels
½ teaspoon garlic powder
½ teaspoon truffle salt
Avocado oil cooking spray or water (see Note)
1 tablespoon chopped fresh parsley leaves, for garnish

1. Pop the popcorn kernels in an air popper or microwave popper according to the manufacturer's instructions or by using the popcorn setting on the microwave.

2. In a small bowl, mix together the garlic powder and truffle salt.

3. Transfer the popcorn to a large bowl and lightly mist it with oil or water. Sprinkle with the seasoning mixture and toss to coat. Garnish with the parsley and serve.

NOTE: You can either mist the popcorn with oil or water. If using water, make sure to use a very light hand, as the popcorn will get soggy easily.

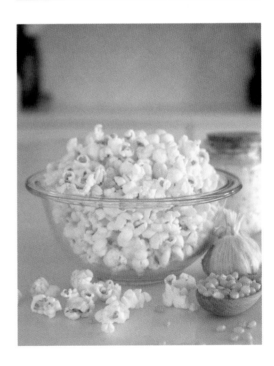

NUTRITION INFORMATION
SERVING SIZE: 1 serving   CALORIES: 164   PROTEIN: 10 g   CARBS: 26 g   FAT: 2 g

Black Bean Salsa

This black bean salsa is delicious served with my baked tortilla chips. For a fun addition/variation, try adding mango or pineapple to it!

1 (15-ounce) can black beans, drained and rinsed

1 (15-ounce) can corn kernels, drained

⅓ cup diced red onion

⅓ cup chopped fresh cilantro leaves

1 medium jalapeño, seeded and diced

Juice of 1 lime

Sea salt

Baked Corn Tortilla Chips (page 210) or sliced cucumbers, for serving

1. In a medium bowl, combine the beans, corn, onion, cilantro, jalapeño, and lime juice. Mix well.

2. Taste and adjust the seasoning with salt, if needed. Enjoy with tortilla chips or cucumber slices. Store leftovers in an airtight container in the refrigerator for up to 5 days.

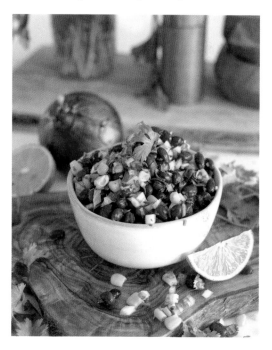

NUTRITION INFORMATION
SERVING SIZE: ½ cup **CALORIES:** 77 **PROTEIN:** 4 g **CARBS:** 11 g **FAT:** 1 g

Pizza

MAKES
4
10-INCH PIZZAS

Friday night is pizza night in my house. It just doesn't seem like the weekend if pizza doesn't make an appearance. I like making my pizza at home with these wholesome ingredients to help me save the fat and calories you get from a restaurant pie. It not only helps me stay on track with my health goals but also helps me feel like I'm not missing out on the weekend yumminess. I love topping mine with onion, bell pepper, mushrooms, olives, artichoke, and cheese sauce! Once it's out of the oven, I always sprinkle a little arugula on top for the peppery bite it gives.

FOR THE ROASTED VEGGIES
16 ounces white mushrooms, sliced
2 red bell peppers, sliced
1 cup chopped broccoli florets
1 medium red onion, sliced
¼ teaspoon garlic salt

FOR THE DOUGH
3½ cups whole wheat flour, plus more for dusting
1 tablespoon instant yeast
2 teaspoons garlic powder
¼ teaspoon sea salt
½ cup unsweetened applesauce, store-bought or homemade
1 cup warm water, plus more if needed
Cornmeal, for dusting

TOPPINGS
4 cups low-fat or oil-free marinara
2 (14-ounce) cans artichoke hearts, drained

¼ cup pitted black olives (optional)
4 cups packed spinach leaves
2 cups Cheese Sauce (page 176), warmed

1. **Make the roasted veggies:** Preheat the oven to 425°F. Line a baking sheet with parchment paper.

2. Spread the mushrooms, bell peppers, broccoli, and onion over the prepared baking sheet. Season with the garlic salt and roast for 25 minutes, or until the vegetables are tender. Set aside to cool; leave the oven on.

3. **While the vegetables are roasting, make the dough:** In the bowl of a stand mixer fitted with the paddle attachment, combine the flour, yeast, garlic powder, and salt. Add the applesauce and mix until combined. With the mixer running on medium speed, slowly add the warm water. If the dough is still dry and crumbly, add more warm water 1 tablespoon at a time until it comes together. Switch to the dough hook and knead the dough on medium speed for 5 to 10 minutes, until it is elastic and firm to the touch. Form the dough into a ball and return it to the mixer bowl. Cover and let stand at room temperature for 20 to 30 minutes, until the dough has doubled in size.

4. Sprinkle a pizza stone or baking sheet with cornmeal. Lightly flour a clean work surface and turn out the dough. Use a rolling pin to roll the dough into a 10-inch round, then carefully transfer it to the prepared pizza stone or pan.

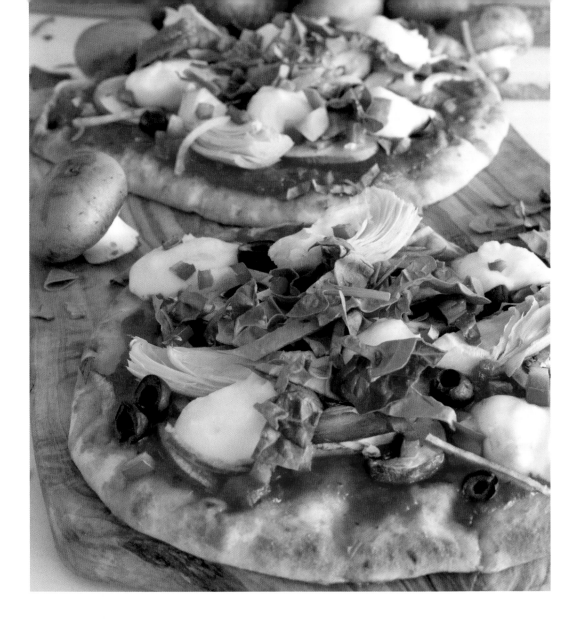

5. Bake the crust for 10 minutes, then remove from the oven and top with the marinara sauce, roasted vegetables, artichokes, and olives (if using). Return the pizza to the oven and bake for 25 minutes, or until the crust is crispy and the center is cooked through. Add the spinach, top with the cheese sauce, and serve.

NOTE: Choose a marinara sauce with 2½ grams of fat or fewer per ½ cup. If you don't have a stand mixer, you can make the dough in a large bowl with a spoon and knead by hand.

NUTRITION INFORMATION
SERVING SIZE: ¼ pizza (without olives) **CALORIES:** 619 **PROTEIN:** 26 g **CARBS:** 100 g **FAT:** 7 g

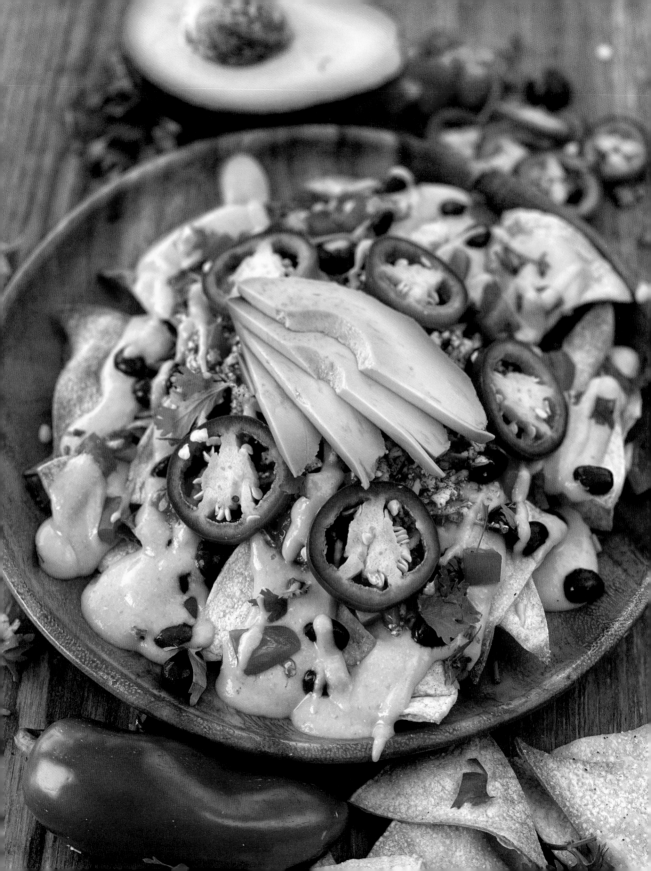

Nachos

SERVES
2

These crunchy baked tortilla chips topped with my cheese sauce and chili-spiced cauliflower, make the perfect craving hitting combo! The cauliflower adds a nice, meaty bite without adding all the extra fat and calories. I love adding salsa, jalapeño slices, and a little avocado! To take these up a step further, try topping them with my cashew sour cream.

---

6 (6-inch) corn tortillas

Sea salt

1 cup riced cauliflower

1 teaspoon chili powder

½ cup cooked or canned black beans or pinto beans (drained and rinsed, if canned)

1 cup Cheese Sauce (page 176), warmed

½ cup chopped tomatoes

½ medium avocado, diced or sliced

2 medium jalapeños, seeded and sliced, or ¼ cup jarred pickled jalapeños (optional)

2 tablespoons Cashew Sour Cream (page 187)

¼ cup salsa, store-bought or homemade (optional)

¼ cup finely chopped fresh cilantro leaves

---

1. Preheat the oven 375°F. Line a baking sheet with parchment paper.

2. Cut the tortillas into chip-size triangles and spread them over the prepared baking sheet. Season with a little salt, if desired, and bake for 8 to 10 minutes, until golden and crisp. Be sure to keep an eye on these—they can go from golden to burned quickly.

3. In a nonstick pan over medium heat, cook the cauliflower until it softens, 3 to 5 minutes. (Alternatively, leave the cauliflower raw.) Season the cauliflower with the chili powder.

4. Arrange the chips on a large plate. Top with the cauliflower, beans, and cheese sauce. Sprinkle with the tomatoes, avocado, jalapeños (if using), sour cream, salsa (if using), and cilantro, then serve.

NOTE: You can choose to steam the cauliflower before seasoning it or just enjoy it raw.

NUTRITION INFORMATION
SERVINGS: 1 serving   **CALORIES:** 421   **PROTEIN:** 13 g   **CARBS:** 55 g   **FAT:** 11 g

Macaroni and Cheese

SERVES

4 OR 5

My favorite childhood meal was always macaroni and cheese—in all its forms! Whether it was from a box or homemade, I was all over it. When I switched to a plant-based diet, this was one of the first dishes I developed for my new lifestyle. I admit, it's not a fancy dish, but honestly, nothing is as delicious or reminiscent of good old mac as simply adding hot cheese sauce to cooked noodles and seasoning with just salt and pepper! For something a little stepped up and more nutritious, add broccoli, mushrooms, or—one of my favorite additions—jalapeños! Dress up this comfort dish any way you like.

1 (12-ounce) box macaroni noodles
(gluten-free or regular)

1 cup plus 2 tablespoons
Cheese Sauce (page 176), warmed

Garlic salt or sea salt

Freshly ground black pepper

1. Cook the pasta according to the package instructions and drain.

2. Return the pasta to the pot and toss with the cheese sauce. Season with garlic salt or salt and pepper. Serve warm.

NUTRITION INFORMATION
SERVING SIZE: 1 cup   **CALORIES:** 340   **PROTEIN:** 12 g   **CARBS:** 62 g   **FAT:** 3 g

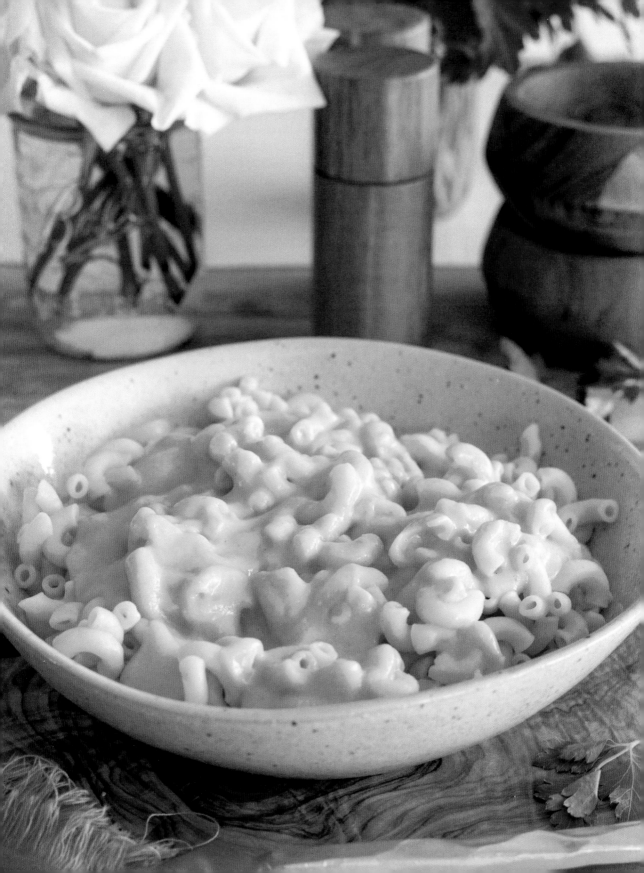

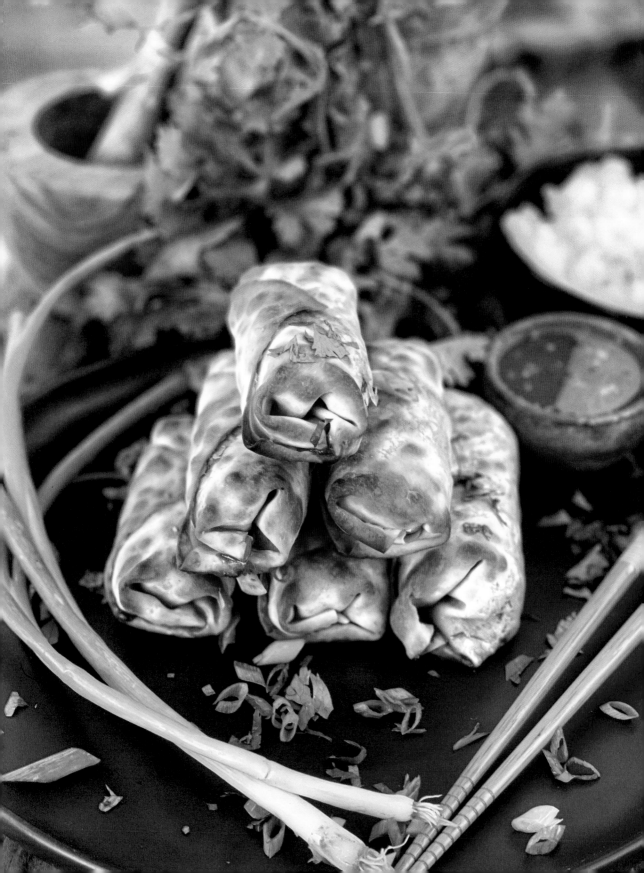

⁵⁰∕₅₀ Egg Rolls

If you're craving Chinese takeout, look no further. These egg rolls could not be easier to make, and they're just as crispy and satisfying as the takeout version—maybe even more crispy, because you're eating them hot, right out of the oven, not from a plastic container! I like serving these with sweet chili sauce. And try pairing them with Chinese Rice and Vegetables (page 85) or Eggless Egg Drop Soup (page 141) for a healthy "Chinese Takeout Night."

2 cups finely shredded napa cabbage

8 ounces white mushrooms, chopped

½ cup diced yellow onion

3 tablespoons low-sodium soy sauce

1 green onion, white and green parts thinly sliced

¼ cup chopped fresh cilantro leaves (optional)

¼ teaspoon toasted sesame oil (optional; see Note)

Chili flakes (optional)

7 vegan egg roll wrappers (I like Nasoya)

Avocado oil cooking spray (optional)

Store-bought sweet chili sauce, for dipping (optional)

1. Preheat the oven to 425°F. Line a baking sheet with parchment paper. (Alternatively, preheat your air fryer.)

2. In a large pot or sauté pan with a fitted lid, combine the cabbage, mushrooms, onion, and soy sauce. Cover and cook over medium-high heat until the vegetables release their liquid, about 10 minutes. Remove the lid and cook for 5 to 10 minutes, until most of the liquid has evaporated. Remove from the heat and stir in the green onion and cilantro, if using. Sprinkle with the sesame oil and some chili flakes if you want heat and mix well.

3. Lay one of the egg roll wrappers on a clean work surface. Scoop ¼ cup of the filling into the center of the wrapper, then roll up the wrapper around the filling like a mini burrito. Place the egg roll on the prepared baking sheet or a plate (if air-frying) and repeat to fill the remaining wrappers.

4. Lightly coat the rolls with avocado oil, if desired (this will help them crisp up, but is not necessary). If using an air fryer, transfer the egg rolls to the basket. Bake or air-fry for 15 to 20 minutes, until the wrappers are golden brown. Let cool slightly before serving (the filling gets hot!), with sweet chili sauce on the side for dipping, if you like.

NOTE: The toasted sesame oil is optional, but it gives these even more flavor and adds just 10 calories and 1 gram of fat to the entire recipe.

NUTRITION INFORMATION
SERVING SIZE: 3½ egg rolls (with sesame oil)   **CALORIES:** 286   **PROTEIN:** 14 g   **CARBS:** 50 g   **FAT:** 1 g

"Crab" Rangoon

MAKES

6

WONTONS

I've never met a person who isn't obsessed with crab rangoon! They're out-of-this-world delicious, and so I wanted to take a swing at remaking them in a healthy, plant-based way. These are every bit as good as the restaurant ones, and are great with Chinese Rice and Vegetables (page 85) and Eggless Egg Drop Soup (page 141) for a Chinese takeout night!

1 cup raw unsalted cashews, soaked overnight (see Note)

2 teaspoons fresh lemon juice

½ teaspoon sea salt, plus more as needed

½ teaspoon garlic powder

¼ teaspoon onion powder

Pinch of chili flakes (optional)

2 tablespoons green onion, white and green parts thinly sliced

6 vegan wonton wrappers (I like Nasoya)

Avocado oil cooking spray (optional)

1. Preheat the oven to 425°F. Line a baking sheet with parchment paper. (Alternatively, preheat your air fryer.)

2. Drain and rinse the cashews and place them in a blender. Add the lemon juice, salt, garlic powder, onion powder, and chili flakes (if using). Pour in ½ cup water and blend until smooth. Use a spoon to fold in the green onion.

3. Lay a few wonton wrappers on a clean work surface and have a small bowl of water nearby. Spoon 1½ teaspoons of the filling into the center of each wrapper. Dampen your index finger with the water and use it to wet the edges of each wrapper. Bring the edges together in a star pattern and press them together to seal. Set the assembled wontons on the prepared baking sheet or a plate (if air-frying) and repeat to fill the remaining wrappers.

4. Lightly spray the wontons with avocado oil, if desired (this will help them get crispy but is not required). If using an air fryer, transfer the wontons to the basket. Bake or air-fry for 15 minutes, or until crispy. Serve immediately by themselves or enjoy with some sweet chili sauce for dipping.

NOTE: If you forget to soak the nuts overnight, just put them in a bowl, pour boiling water over them, and let them soak for 4 hours. This will soften them enough to blend smoothly.

NUTRITION INFORMATION
SERVING SIZE: 3 wontons   **CALORIES:** 142   **PROTEIN:** 5 g   **CARBS:** 16 g   **FAT:** 7 g

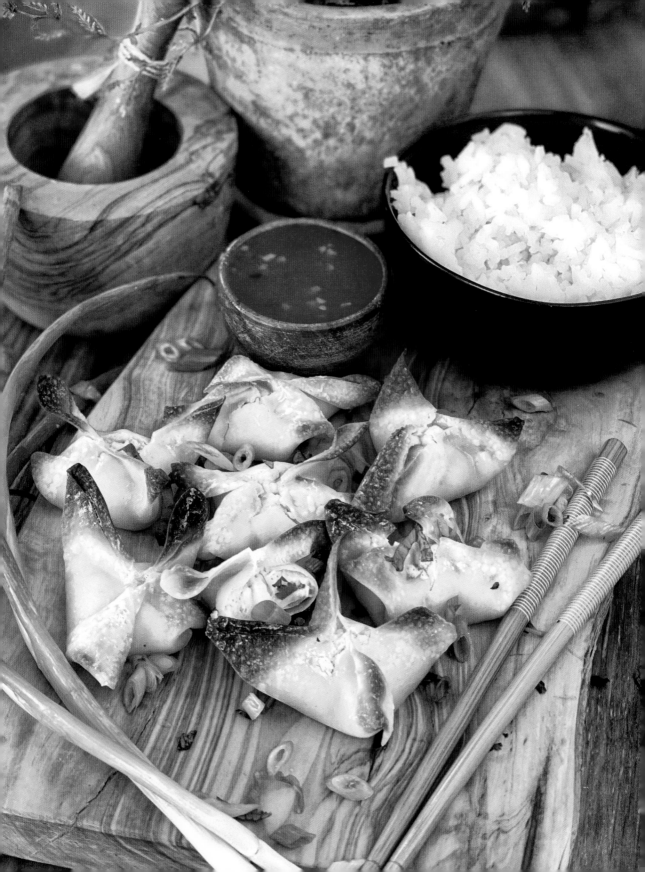

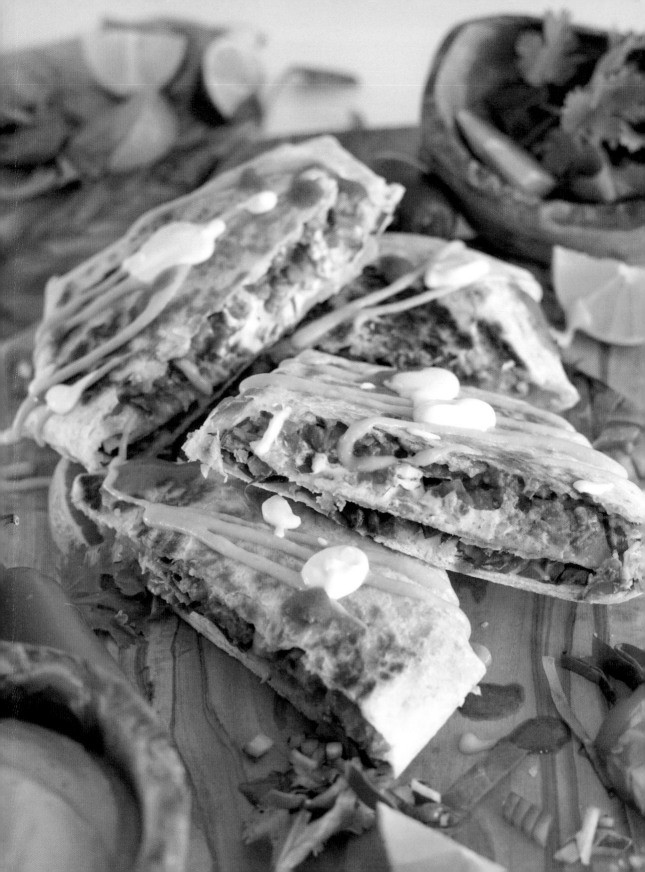

Crunchy Tostada Wrap

MAKES
2
WRAPS

I used to have a Mexican fast-food problem . . . a bad one! I loved Mexican takeout with a passion, so I knew that without an alternative, so much of my effort to get healthy and lose weight would be compromised by the challenge of giving it up. Luckily, these wraps are everything I needed them to be: crispy, gooey, and filling. They're a fan favorite in my family, and we love topping them with our favorite hot sauce. I sometimes buy Taco Bell hot sauce at the store, for old times' sake—it's oil-free!

FOR THE LENTIL TACO "MEAT"

¼ cup diced yellow onion

½ cup canned brown lentils, drained

1 tablespoon taco seasoning

TO ASSEMBLE

2 (6-inch) corn tortillas

½ cup fat-free refried beans, homemade or store-bought

½ cup Cheese Sauce (page 176), warmed

¼ cup Cashew Sour Cream (page 187), plus more for serving

2 Roma (plum) tomatoes, diced

1 cup chopped romaine lettuce

Your favorite hot sauce (optional)

2 (10-inch) flour tortillas (see Note)

1. Preheat the oven to 400°F.

2. **Make the taco "meat":** In a large nonstick sauté pan, cook the onion over medium-high heat until just softened, 1 to 2 minutes. Add the lentils, taco seasoning, and 2 tablespoons water and mix well. Remove the pan from the heat once the lentils are hot and set aside.

3. **Assemble the tostadas:** Arrange the corn tortillas on a baking sheet and toast in the oven until crisp, 8 minutes. Remove from the oven and layer the toasted tortillas with the lentil mixture, refried beans, cheese sauce, sour cream, tomatoes, lettuce, and hot sauce, if desired.

4. Heat a large nonstick sauté pan over medium-high heat. Place a tostada in the center of a flour tortilla and fold the edges of the flour tortilla toward the center to completely enclose the tostada. Carefully place the wrapped tostada in the pan, folded-side down, and sear for 3 to 5 minutes, until golden brown. Flip and cook for 3 to 5 minutes on the second side, then transfer to a plate. Repeat with the remaining tostada and flour tortilla.

5. Serve with additional sour cream and hot sauce, if desired.

> **NOTE:** You'll use both corn tortillas and flour tortillas in this recipe—try to find flour tortillas that are as low in fat as possible. I like the Olé Mexican Foods Xtreme Wellness tortillas or wraps.

NUTRITION INFORMATION
SERVING SIZE: 1 wrap   **CALORIES:** 353   **PROTEIN:** 19 g   **CARBS:** 42 g   **FAT:** 9 g

Onion Rings

MAKES
18
ONION RINGS

Onion rings are, not surprisingly, at the top of my craving must-haves list! With salt, onion powder, and a bread crumb coating, they're crunchy and delicious, and in no way need to be fried to be amazing. Sometimes I'll make a meal of just onion rings—I'm not ashamed to admit it!

½ cup whole wheat flour, oat flour, or rice flour

¼ teaspoon sea salt

¼ teaspoon garlic powder, plus more as needed

¼ teaspoon onion powder

Ground black pepper

1 cup panko bread crumbs (gluten-free or regular)

1 large Vidalia onion, sliced into ½-inch-thick rings (about 18)

Ketchup, for serving (optional)

1. Preheat the oven or an air fryer to 425°F. Line a baking sheet with parchment paper.

2. In a medium bowl, whisk together the flour, salt, garlic powder, onion powder, and a pinch of pepper. While whisking, slowly add ½ cup water and whisk until well combined. Place the bread crumbs in a shallow dish and set them next to the batter.

3. Working with one at a time, dip an onion ring into the batter to coat, allowing any excess to drip off, then dredge it in the panko. Place the battered onion ring on the prepared baking sheet and repeat to coat the remaining onion.

4. Bake for 15 to 20 minutes in the oven or 12 to 15 minutes in the air fryer, until golden and crispy. If you like, season the onion rings with more garlic salt, then enjoy with ketchup, if desired.

NUTRITION INFORMATION
SERVING SIZE: 9 onion rings **CALORIES:** 256 **PROTEIN:** 8 g **CARBS:** 52 g **FAT:** 0.5 g

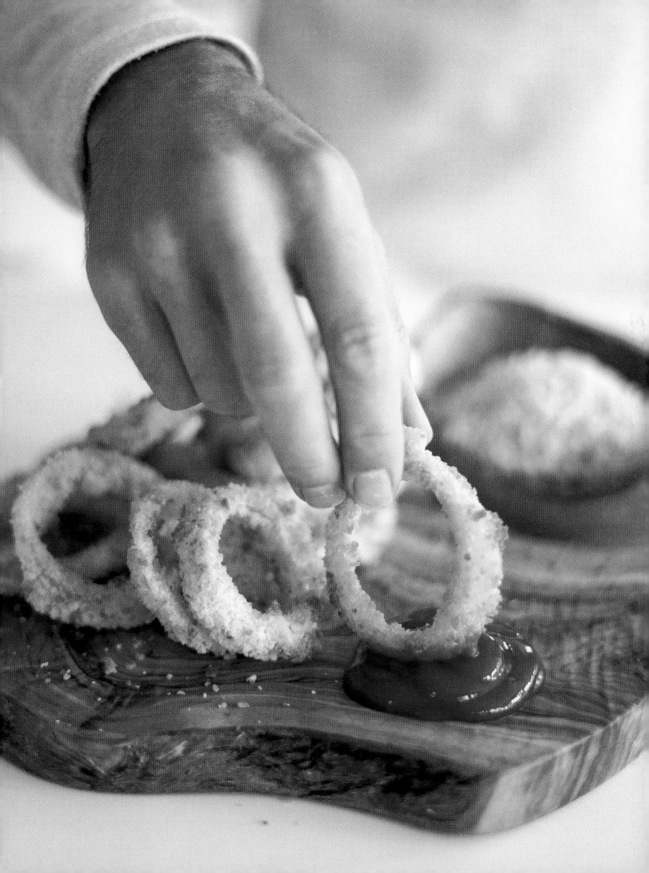

CHAPTER 5

Desserts

Mini Oat Bar Bites

Sometimes you just need a little bite of something sweet, and these mini oat bars deliver. I use powdered peanut butter to help keep them oil free. If you want to further reduce the calories, use all-natural sugar-free maple syrup or stevia to sweeten. These keep well in an airtight container in the freezer for up to two weeks.

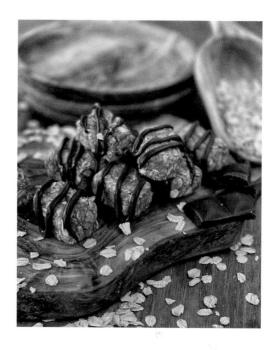

½ cup powdered peanut butter (I like PB2)

1 tablespoon pure maple syrup

½ teaspoon pure vanilla extract

1 cup rolled oats

2 tablespoons dairy-free chocolate chips, melted (I like Enjoy Life vegan mini chocolate chips)

1. In a medium bowl, stir together the powdered peanut butter, maple syrup, and vanilla. Add the oats and ¼ cup water and mix well.

2. Use a tablespoon to scoop the mixture into your hands and form it into small bars. Arrange the bars on a baking sheet and drizzle with the chocolate. Let the chocolate set for 10 minutes, then store the bars in an airtight container in the refrigerator for up to 5 days.

NUTRITION INFORMATION
SERVING SIZE: 2 bars   CALORIES: 132   PROTEIN: 6 g   CARBS: 16 g   FAT: 4 g

Berries with Chocolate Chips

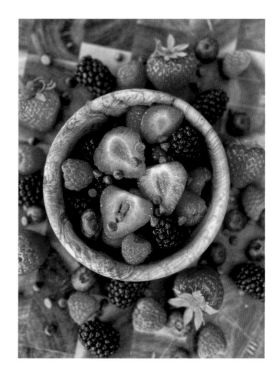

When you're trying to cut back on unhealthy evening snacking (you know, the snacking that happens after dinner when you're watching your favorite show), berries and chocolate are surprisingly satisfying. Strawberries are extremely nutrient-dense (vitamin C, folates, and potassium!) and super low in calories, and when topped with some vegan chocolate, they make a great evening dessert. If you can't find dairy-free chocolate chips, opt for some chocolate sprinkles! They're usually dairy-free and even lower in calories than chocolate chips.

4 cups fresh strawberries, hulled and sliced, or mixed berries

1 tablespoon dairy-free mini chocolate chips (I like Enjoy Life vegan mini chocolate chips)

Divide the berries between two bowls, top with the chocolate chips, and serve.

NUTRITION INFORMATION
SERVING SIZE: 1 serving   **CALORIES:** 137   **PROTEIN:** 3 g   **CARBS:** 221 g   **FAT:** 3 g

Caramel Apple Streusel

MAKES
2
STREUSELS

My husband came up with this dessert one night when he was scrounging around the kitchen looking for something sweet. All we had in the fridge were a few apples and a few dates. He intelligently crafted this decadent, comforting dessert all on his own—I can take no credit for it other than adding the maple syrup drizzle at the end.

1 Honeycrisp apple, cored

4 Medjool dates, pitted

Ground cinnamon

2 tablespoons Weight Loss–Friendly Granola (page 206)

1 teaspoon pure maple syrup (optional)

1. Preheat the oven to 425°F. Line a baking sheet with parchment paper. (Alternatively, you can make this dish in the microwave.)

2. Using a mandoline or a sharp knife, slice the apple as thinly as possible; try to get 10 slices or so. Lay 1 slice on the preparing baking sheet (or on a microwave-safe plate, if microwaving) and spread ½ date over the top. Top with another apple slice, followed by a small pinch of cinnamon. Repeat to make three additional layers, ending with apple on top; this is 1 streusel. Use the remaining apples, dates, and cinnamon to make a second streusel.

3. Bake the streusels for 6 minutes or microwave for 1 minute, until the apples are warmed through. Transfer each streusel to a plate and top with the granola and the maple syrup, if desired.

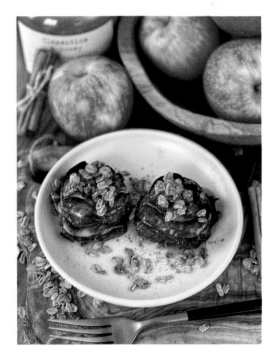

NUTRITION INFORMATION
SERVING SIZE: 1 streusel **CALORIES:** 209 **PROTEIN:** 2 g **CARBS:** 49 g **FAT:** 1 g

Candy Bar Bites

I don't know a single person who doesn't love a good candy bar. And if you've never had the magical combination of dates, chocolate, and peanut butter . . . you're in for a treat! These make great gifts and are even better refrigerated, as they become chewy like a caramel.

---

2 tablespoons powdered peanut butter (I like PB2)

6 Medjool dates, pitted

1 tablespoon dairy-free mini chocolate chips (I like Enjoy Life vegan mini chocolate chips) or chocolate sprinkles (see Note)

---

1. In a small bowl, stir together the powdered peanut butter and 1 tablespoon plus 1 teaspoon water. Transfer the peanut butter to a small plastic sandwich bag and use scissors to snip off one of the corners.

2. Arrange the dates on a plate and pipe a drizzle of the peanut butter over them. Top with the chocolate chips or sprinkles and enjoy. Store leftovers in an airtight container in the refrigerator for up to 1 week.

> **NOTE:** Sprinkles bring plenty of chocolate flavor and add even fewer calories, so feel free to use those instead of chocolate chips.

NUTRITION INFORMATION
SERVING SIZE: 3 pieces   **CALORIES:** 231   **PROTEIN:** 4 g   **CARBS:** 47 g   **FAT:** 3 g

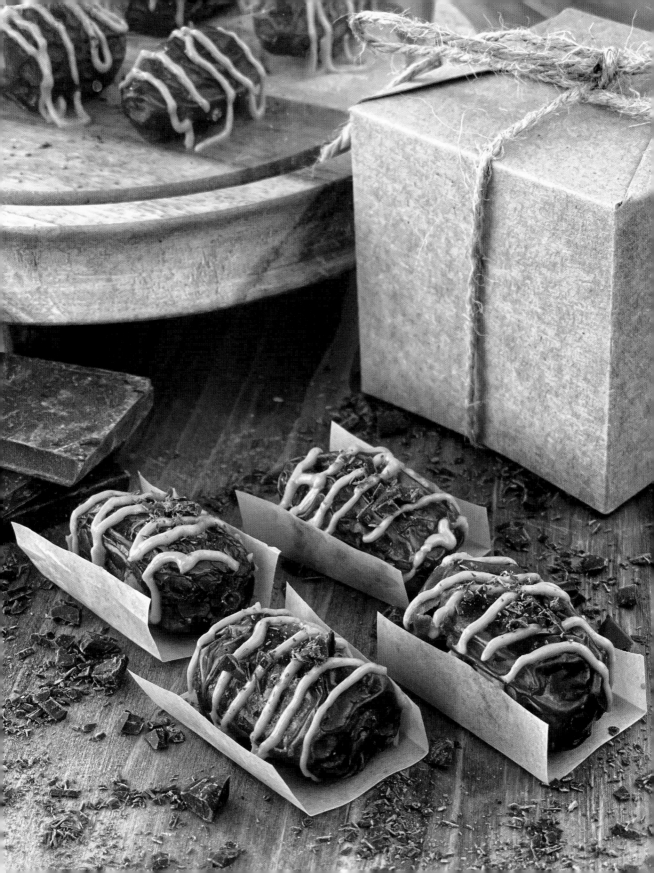

Chocolate "Nice Cream"

I was stunned at how easy making plant-based ice cream can be, and you don't even need a fancy high-speed blender! All you need are a food processor, a few frozen bananas, and a little imagination. This "nice cream" is chocolaty and totally hits the spot. My kids love making this and adding some fun sprinkles!

NOTE: I like using almond milk for this, or use a plant-based milk with around 30 calories per cup.

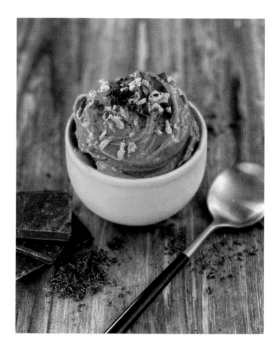

4 medium bananas, peeled and frozen

¼ cup plain, unsweetened plant-based milk (see Note)

3 tablespoons unsweetened cocoa powder

2 teaspoons pure vanilla extract

In a food processor or high-speed blender, combine the bananas, milk, cocoa powder, and vanilla. Process until smooth. Serve immediately or store in a freezer-safe container in the freezer for up to 1 week.

NUTRITION INFORMATION
SERVING SIZE: ½ cup   **CALORIES:** 107   **PROTEIN:** 2 g   **CARBS:** 22 g   **FAT:** 1 g

Chocolate Chip Cookie Dough "Nice Cream"

There's a locally owned ice cream shop called Walrus Ice Cream in Fort Collins, Colorado, that makes the best chocolate chip cookie dough ice cream! They take soft cookie dough and fold it into the ice cream right in front of you, then put it into your cone or cup. This is my plant-based take on that ice cream. Make sure you refrigerate your cookie dough first so it firms up before you try to mix it into your "nice cream."

4 medium bananas, peeled and frozen

¼ cup plain, unsweetened
plant-based milk (see Note on page 234)

2 teaspoons pure vanilla extract

8 tablespoons Chocolate Chip Cookie Dough
(page 246), chilled overnight

1. In a food processor or high-speed blender, combine the bananas, milk, and vanilla. Process until smooth.

2. Top with the cookie dough and serve immediately, or store in a freezer-safe container in the freezer for up to 1 week.

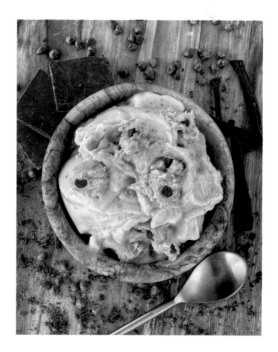

NUTRITION INFORMATION
SERVING SIZE: ½ cup with 2 tablespoons cookie dough   **CALORIES:** 116   **PROTEIN:** 2 g   **CARBS:** 24 g   **FAT:** 1 g

Strawberry Shortcake "Nice Cream"

MAKES

2

CUPS

Of all the "nice creams" in this book, this one is my favorite! The crunch from the granola and sweetness from the strawberries and bananas are perfectly satisfying. I make this one for company, because it always comes out so pretty.

4 medium bananas, peeled and frozen

2½ cups frozen strawberries

¼ cup plain, unsweetened plant-based milk (see Note on page 234)

2 teaspoons pure vanilla extract

2 tablespoons Weight Loss–Friendly Granola (page 206)

1. In a food processor or high-speed blender, combine the bananas, strawberries, milk, and vanilla. Process until mostly smooth; I like to leave some chunks for texture.

2. Top with the granola and serve immediately, or store in a freezer-safe container in the freezer for up to 1 week.

NUTRITION INFORMATION
SERVING SIZE: ½ cup nice cream with 2 tablespoons granola   **CALORIES:** 106   **PROTEIN:** 1 g   **CARBS:** 22 g   **FAT:** 0.5 g

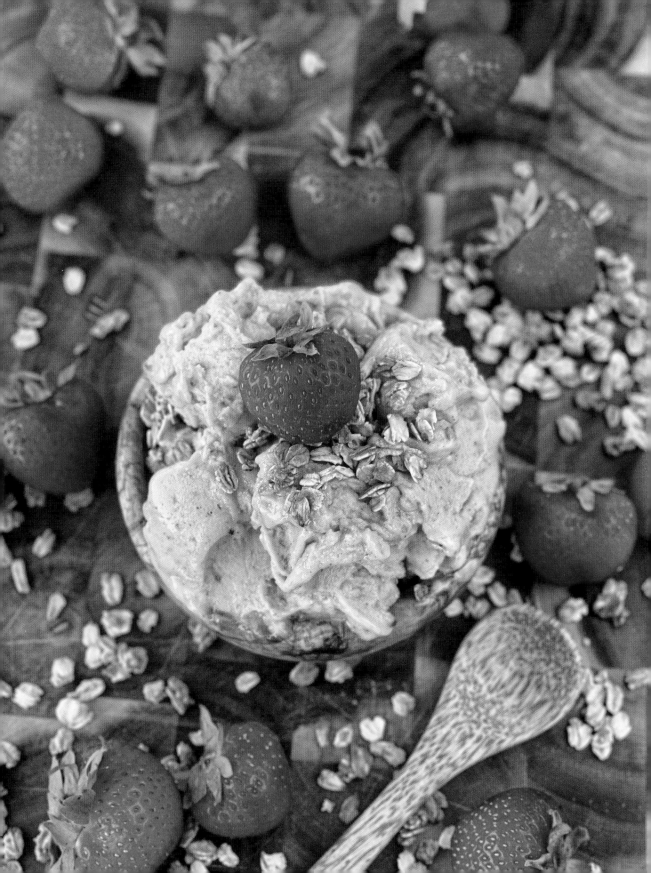

Mint Chocolate Chip "Nice Cream"

Mint is a wonderful way to cleanse the palate—add a little chocolate, and you have a dessert! I love making this Mint Chocolate Chip "Nice Cream." It's cooling and decadent and satisfies my sweet tooth.

4 medium bananas, peeled and frozen

¼ cup plain, unsweetened plant-based milk (see Note on page 234)

1 teaspoon pure vanilla extract

¼ teaspoon mint extract

4 teaspoons dairy-free chocolate chips (I like Enjoy Life vegan mini chocolate chips)

Chocolate sprinkles, for serving (optional)

1. In a food processor or high-speed blender, combine the bananas, milk, vanilla, and mint extract. Process until smooth.

2. Top with the chocolate chips and sprinkles, if desired, then serve immediately, or store in a freezer-safe container in the freezer for up to 1 week.

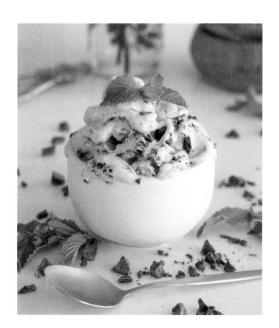

NUTRITION INFORMATION
SERVING SIZE: ½ cup with 1 teaspoon dairy-free chocolate chips   **CALORIES:** 122   **PROTEIN:** 2 g   **CARBS:** 23 g   **FAT:** 2 g

Chocolate Cherry "Nice Cream"

The light sprinkle of walnuts on this "nice cream" makes such a wonderful addition. The cherries and the cocoa powder give it a smooth, decadent flavor.

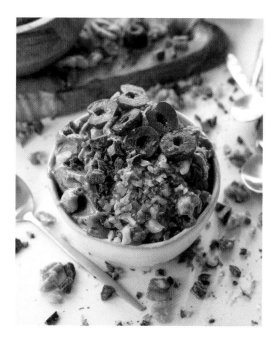

4 medium bananas, peeled and frozen

1 cup frozen cherries

¼ cup plain, unsweetened plant-based milk (see Note on page 234)

2 tablespoons unsweetened cocoa powder

1 teaspoon pure vanilla extract

2 whole walnuts, chopped, for serving

Cocoa nibs, for serving

1. In a food processor or high-speed blender, combine the bananas, cherries, milk, cocoa powder, and vanilla. Process until smooth.

2. Divide the mixture between two bowls and top with the walnuts and cocoa nibs.

NUTRITION INFORMATION
SERVING SIZE: ½ cup   **CALORIES:** 214   **PROTEIN:** 4 g   **CARBS:** 42 g   **FAT:** 2.7 g

Chocolate Pudding and Raspberries

SERVES
2

This chocolate pudding is so easy to whip together and serve over fresh raspberries! The pudding tastes rich and decadent, and the raspberries add a delicious light flavor.

2 cups almond milk (see Note)

2 tablespoons unsweetened cocoa powder

3 tablespoons cornstarch or arrowroot powder

1 teaspoon vanilla extract

Stevia to taste (for stevia drops, use 20 to 30; for powdered stevia, use 2 to 4 tablespoons or to taste)

2 cups raspberries

Cocoa nibs or chocolate sprinkles, for serving (optional)

1. In a medium saucepan, combine the almond milk, cocoa powder, and cornstarch or arrowroot and whisk until the dry ingredients are fully incorporated into the milk and no clumps remain. This will take 1 to 2 minutes of vigorous mixing.

2. Cook the mixture over medium-high heat until it begins to simmer, stirring constantly so the bottom doesn't burn and the pudding is smooth and doesn't clump. Once the mixture has thickened enough to cover the back of a spoon, about 2 to 3 minutes, remove it from the heat.

3. Stir in the vanilla extract and stevia to taste. Allow the mixture to cool in the refrigerator for 20 to 30 minutes and it will thicken up even more.

4. Divide the raspberries between two small bowls and top each with half the pudding. Top with the cocoa nibs or sprinkles, if desired, and enjoy.

NOTE: When preparing the pudding, be sure to use low-calorie almond milk to help save on calories. Look for one around 30 calories per cup.

NUTRITION INFORMATION
SERVING SIZE: 1 serving (without cocoa nibs or sprinkles)   **CALORIES:** 192   **PROTEIN:** 3 g   **CARBS:** 35 g   **FAT:** 2 g

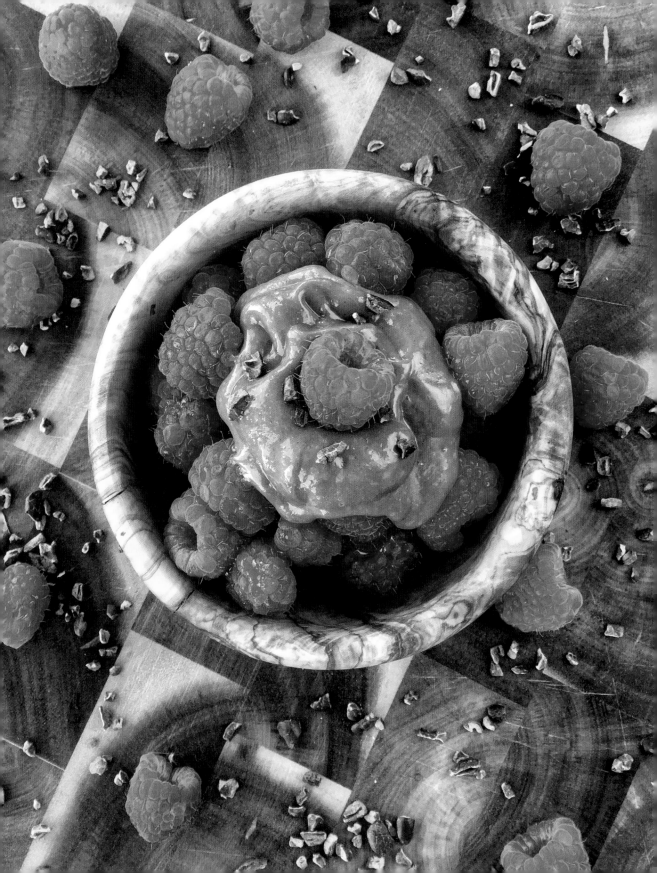

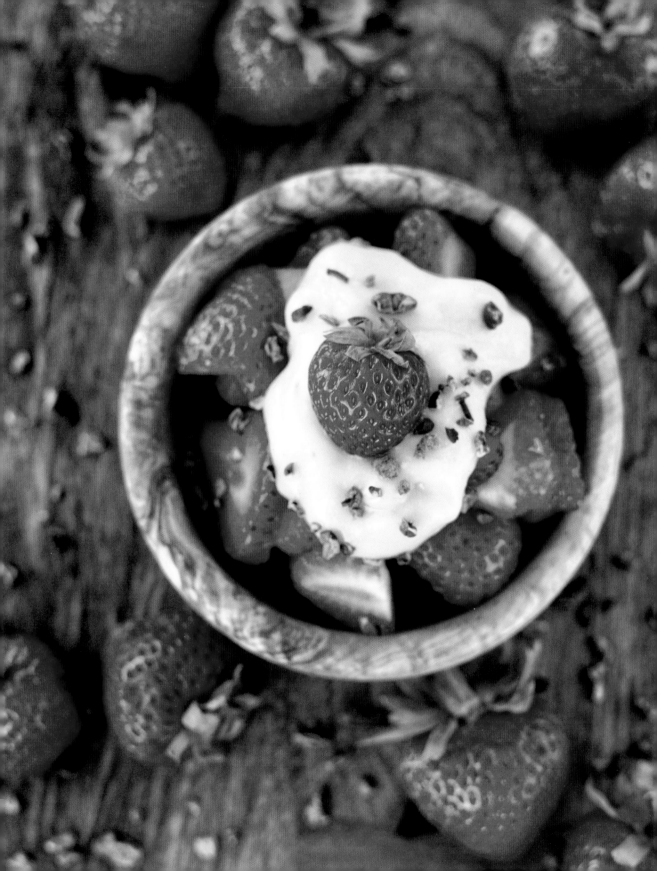

Vanilla Pudding and Strawberries

I've always loved pudding but never realized just how easy it is to make at home—and that it can be made with just a few ingredients, and it's only a handful of calories. I sweeten this pudding with stevia and then add fresh berries to it to make a decadent and satisfying dessert.

---

2 cups almond milk

3 tablespoons cornstarch or arrowroot powder

1 teaspoon vanilla extract

Stevia to taste (for stevia drops, use 20 to 30; for powdered stevia, use 2 to 4 tablespoons or to taste)

2 cups hulled strawberries

Cocoa nibs or chocolate sprinkles, for serving (optional)

---

1. In a medium saucepan, combine the almond milk and cornstarch or arrowroot and whisk until the powder is fully incorporated into the milk and no clumps remain.

2. Cook the mixture over medium-high heat until it begins to simmer, stirring constantly so the bottom doesn't burn and the pudding is smooth and doesn't clump. Once the mixture has thickened enough to cover the back of a spoon, about 2 to 3 minutes, remove it from the heat.

3. Stir in the vanilla extract and stevia to taste. Allow the mixture to cool in the refrigerator for 20 to 30 minutes and it will thicken up even more.

4. Divide the strawberries between two small bowls and top each with half the pudding. Top with the cocoa nibs or sprinkles, if desired, and enjoy.

NUTRITION INFORMATION
SERVING SIZE: 1 serving (without cocoa nibs or sprinkles)   **CALORIES:** 167   **PROTEIN:** 2 g   **CARBS:** 34 g   **FAT:** 2 g

Frozen Fruit Desserts

Frozen fruit makes a great dessert option when you're on your weight loss journey. It is low in calorie density and high in nutrition and fiber, and it has a lot of bulk, which will help satisfy you. I found that adding some sprinkles on top of my frozen fruit gives it a fun crunchy texture and makes it all the more enjoyable.

Frozen Cherries with Cocoa Nibs or Sprinkles

2 cups frozen cherries
2 teaspoons sprinkles or cocoa nibs

Divide the cherries between two bowls and sprinkle with the cocoa nibs or sprinkles, then serve.

NUTRITION INFORMATION
SERVING SIZE: 1 serving   **CALORIES:** 106   **PROTEIN:** 2 g
CARBS: 17 g   **FAT:** 2 g

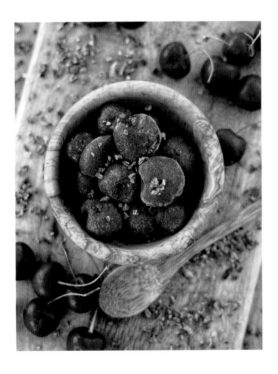

Frozen Blueberries

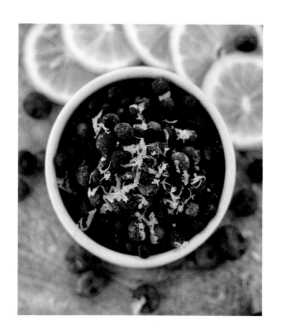

2 cups frozen blueberries

2 teaspoons sprinkles, or ¼ teaspoon lemon zest (or use both!), for topping

Divide the blueberries between two bowls and top evenly with the sprinkles, the lemon zest, or both, then serve.

NUTRITION INFORMATION
SERVING SIZE: 1 serving **CALORIES:** 71 **PROTEIN:** 0.5 g
CARBS: 13 g **FAT:** 2 g

Frozen Pineapple

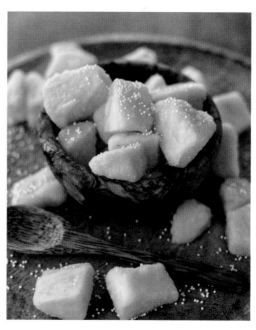

2 cups frozen pineapple

2 teaspoons sprinkles

Divide the pineapple between two bowls and top with the sprinkles, then serve.

NUTRITION INFORMATION
SERVING SIZE: 1 serving **CALORIES:** 108 **PROTEIN:** 1 g
CARBS: 23 g **FAT:** 1 g

Chocolate Chip Cookies

MAKES
1½
CUPS DOUGH
OR 17 COOKIES

When I was growing up, my mom would occasionally buy us a big tub of cookie dough. Anytime my friends and I got a cookie craving, we could scoop some dough onto a baking sheet and have fresh cookies in minutes. But there were plenty of other times when we'd just get into the tub of cookie dough with spoons and eat it right out of the container. So this recipe is dedicated to the many tubs of cookie dough I consumed throughout my childhood. For another craving-satisfying way to enjoy this dough, use it in the Chocolate Chip Cookie Dough "Nice Cream" (page 235), or bake it as cookies to enjoy warm from the oven.

1 (15-ounce) can chickpeas, drained and rinsed

¼ cup pure maple syrup

2 teaspoons pure vanilla extract

½ teaspoon baking powder

¼ cup oat flour

Pinch of sea salt

2 tablespoons dairy-free mini chocolate chips (I like Enjoy Life vegan mini chocolate chips)

1. In a food processor or high-speed blender, combine the chickpeas, maple syrup, vanilla extract, baking powder, oat flour, and sea salt. Process until smooth, then transfer to a bowl and stir in the chocolate chips.

2. To bake it into cookies, preheat the oven to 375°F. Line a baking sheet with parchment paper.

3. Use a tablespoon to portion the dough onto the prepared baking sheet, leaving about 2 inches between each. Gently flatten each ball of dough and bake for 13 minutes, or until the cookies are slightly puffed but not dried out. Allow them to cool in the pan.

4. Store the cookies in a freezer-safe container in the freezer for up to 1 month—that way, you're not tempted to snack on them all at once!

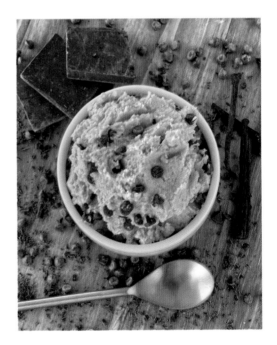

NUTRITION INFORMATION

SERVING SIZE: ¼ cup dough   **CALORIES:** 141   **PROTEIN:** 4 g   **CARBS:** 21 g   **FAT:** 3 g

SERVING SIZE: 4 cookies   **CALORIES:** 199   **PROTEIN:** 6 g   **CARBS:** 30 g   **FAT:** 4 g

Chocolate Lava Cake

As a woman I can fully attest to the fact that chocolate is a need, not a want … and as such, I would never ask anyone to remove chocolate from their diet—I can think of nothing worse! This little mug cake has saved me many times when a chocolate craving hits. It also makes a great easy dessert if you have unexpected company stop by.

2 tablespoons whole wheat flour, oat flour, or gluten-free flour

1 tablespoon unrefined sugar

2 tablespoons dairy-free mini chocolate chips (I like Enjoy Life vegan mini chocolate chips)

1 tablespoon unsweetened cocoa powder

¼ teaspoon baking powder

⅛ teaspoon sea salt

2 tablespoons unsweetened plant-based milk

1 tablespoon unsweetened applesauce, homemade or store-bought

½ teaspoon pure vanilla extract (see Note)

Confectioners' sugar, for garnish (optional)

1. Divide the flour, sugar, chocolate chips, cocoa powder, baking powder, and salt between two 4-ounce ramekins or put into a small mug. Mix well. Stir in the milk, applesauce, and vanilla.

2. Microwave the ramekins or the mug for 40 seconds for a gooier cake or 50 seconds for a firmer cake. Dust the top with confectioners' sugar, if you like, and enjoy.

NOTE: I call for ½ teaspoon pure vanilla extract in this recipe because I love its flavor, but my husband prefers less, about ¼ teaspoon. Feel free to adjust the measurement to your liking!

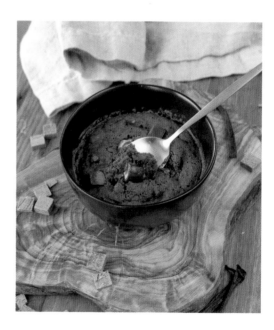

NUTRITION INFORMATION
SERVING SIZE: 1 cake   CALORIES: 295   PROTEIN: 5 g   CARBS: 42 g   FAT: 11 g

Gluten-Free Oat Cinnamon Rolls

MAKES
8
CINNAMON
ROLLS

There's a little diner called the Silver Grill in the town where I grew up that's known for its enormous and delicious cinnamon rolls. It was always a special treat to go to the Silver Grill on Saturday mornings for breakfast, during which the warm, fresh rolls played the starring part. I think that's where my love affair with cinnamon rolls started. My version swaps all the fat and sugar of a standard cinnamon roll for gluten-free oats, dates, and natural sweetener, and not only do they taste just as good, they won't leave you full one minute and then coming down from a sugar high the next. And best of all, they come together quickly.

Avocado oil cooking spray (optional)

FOR THE FILLING
1 cup Medjool dates, pitted
½ Fuji apple, cored and diced
¼ cup pure maple syrup
1 teaspoon ground cinnamon
½ teaspoon pure vanilla extract

FOR THE DOUGH
3 cups oat flour
⅓ cup unrefined sugar or coconut sugar (optional; see Note)
2 teaspoons baking powder
½ teaspoon sea salt
2 teaspoons pure vanilla extract

½ cup confectioners' sugar, for glazing (optional)

1. Preheat the oven to 375°F. Line a baking sheet with parchment paper or lightly coat a nonstick baking pan with avocado oil.

2. **Make the filling:** In a blender or food processor, combine the dates, apple, maple syrup, cinnamon, and vanilla. Blend until smooth and set aside.

3. **Make the dough:** In a large bowl, combine the flour, sugar (if using), baking powder, and salt. Stir to mix well.

4. In a medium bowl, combine the vanilla with 1 cup water and mix well. While stirring slowly, pour the vanilla mixture into the dry ingredients and mix until an even dough forms. At first it will seem like there's not enough water, but keep mixing! This will not be wet like a muffin batter, but it will be sticky.

5. Turn out the dough onto a piece of waxed paper. Wet your hands, then shape the dough into a rectangle. Place a second piece of waxed paper on top of the dough and use a rolling pin to roll it out to ¼ to ½ inch thick. Gently peel off the top piece of waxed paper and discard. Spoon the filling over the dough and use a knife or spatula to spread it into an even layer.

6. Beginning from one of the short ends of the rectangle, roll up the dough. This can be a little tricky, but after a few tries, you'll get it. Carefully slice the roll crosswise into 8 even pieces and arrange

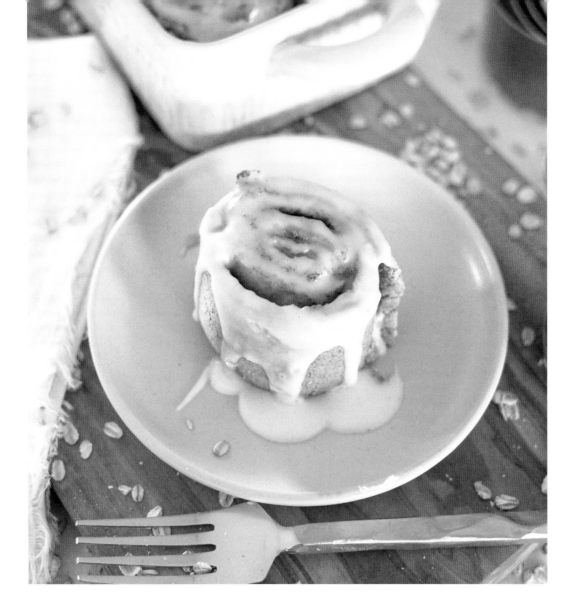

them cut side down on the prepared pan. They may not hold their shape perfectly, but they will taste amazing.

7. Bake for 20 to 25 minutes, until the cinnamon rolls are set but not drying out. Remove from the oven and let cool slightly.

8. Meanwhile, if you'd like to glaze the rolls, mix together the confectioners' sugar and 2 teaspoons water in a small bowl until smooth. Drizzle the rolls with the glaze while they're still warm. Store any leftovers in an airtight container for up to 2 days.

NUTRITION INFORMATION
SERVING SIZE: 1 glazed roll   **CALORIES:** 332   **PROTEIN:** 6 g   **CARBS:** 65 g   **FAT:** 3 g

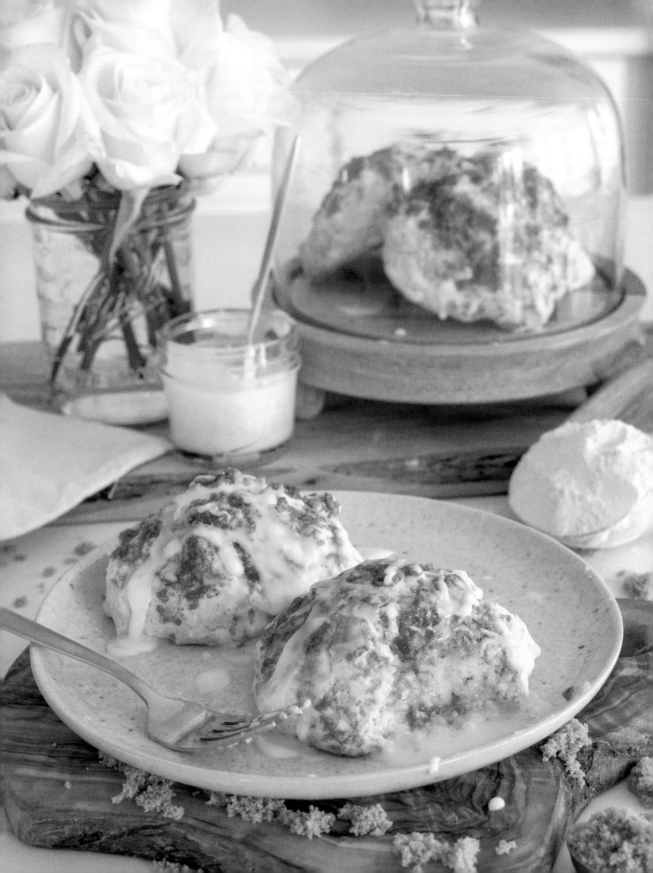

Easy Cinnamon Roll Biscuits

These biscuits are for those of us who love cinnamon rolls but not the time and effort they require in the kitchen. They taste like cinnamon rolls, but because they're biscuits, they're easy to throw together. These are great for satisfying a dessert craving, and I'm pretty sure anyone else in your house will enjoy them as well!

FOR THE TOPPING
¼ cup packed brown sugar
1 teaspoon pure vanilla extract
½ teaspoon ground cinnamon

FOR THE BISCUITS
2 cups whole wheat flour
2 teaspoons baking powder
½ teaspoon ground cinnamon
½ teaspoon sea salt

¼ cup confectioners' sugar, for glazing (optional)

1. Preheat the oven to 375°F. Line a baking sheet with parchment paper.

2. **Make the topping:** In a small bowl, stir together the brown sugar, vanilla, and cinnamon. Set aside.

3. **Make the biscuits:** In a medium bowl, stir together the flour, baking powder, cinnamon, and salt. While stirring, slowly add 1¼ cups water and stir until just combined. You want the batter to be clumpy, not runny. If the batter is dry and crumbly, try adding more water 1 tablespoon at a time; you most likely won't need more than another ¼ cup.

4. Using a ¼-cup scoop, drop the batter in mounds on the prepared baking sheet. Divide the topping among the biscuits and bake for 15 to 20 minutes, until starting to brown. Remove from the oven and let cool slightly.

5. Meanwhile, if you'd like to glaze the biscuits, mix together the confectioners' sugar and 1 teaspoon water in a small bowl until smooth. The glaze should be thin enough to drizzle. If needed, add 1 more teaspoon of water.

6. Drizzle the biscuits with the glaze and serve warm. You can store leftovers in an airtight container on the counter for 2 days.

NUTRITION INFORMATION
SERVING SIZE: 2 biscuits drizzled with glaze   **CALORIES:** 358   **PROTEIN:** 9 g   **CARBS:** 64 g   **FAT:** 5 g

Black Bean Brownies

MAKES
9
BROWNIES

The thought of black beans in brownies may seem unusual, but hear me out. After I committed to a low-fat diet, I tried baking brownies without butter or oil, but I couldn't get that fudgy brownie texture. Without the fat, they ended up more like cake than brownies. It turns out that black beans give you that fudgy texture, without having to add oil or vegan butter! You can't taste the beans themselves, and you're getting the added benefit of their protein, fiber, and other nutrients. It's a win-win!

---

2 (15-ounce) cans black beans, drained and rinsed

½ cup unsweetened cocoa powder

½ cup whole wheat flour (see Note)

½ cup unsweetened applesauce, homemade or store-bought

½ cup pure maple syrup

3 tablespoons powdered vegan egg replacer (I like Bob's Red Mill) or tapioca flour

2 teaspoons pure vanilla extract

1 teaspoon baking powder

½ teaspoon sea salt

½ cup dairy-free mini chocolate chips (I like Enjoy Life vegan mini chocolate chips)

---

1. Preheat the oven to 375°F. In a food processor, combine the beans, cocoa powder, flour, applesauce, maple syrup, egg replacer, vanilla, baking powder, and salt. Process until completely smooth.

2. Scrape the batter into an 8-inch square silicone baking pan that has been placed on a baking sheet for stability. Use a spatula or wooden spoon to fold in the chocolate chips, or simply sprinkle them on top of the batter. Bake for 30 to 35 minutes, until the brownies are set but still soft. They should be fudgy. Let cool slightly, then slice into 9 even pieces and serve. Store leftover brownies in an airtight container in the refrigerator for up to 5 days.

> **NOTE:** Feel free to use gluten-free flour instead. I like Bob's Red Mill Gluten-Free 1-to-1 Baking Flour. Also, I call for baking the brownies in a silicone pan, which I love because you don't have to grease it first. That said, you can use a regular baking pan instead—just lightly coat it with avocado oil cooking spray before adding the batter.

NUTRITION INFORMATION
SERVING SIZE: 1 brownie **CALORIES:** 249 **PROTEIN:** 8 g **CARBS:** 37 g **FAT:** 6 g

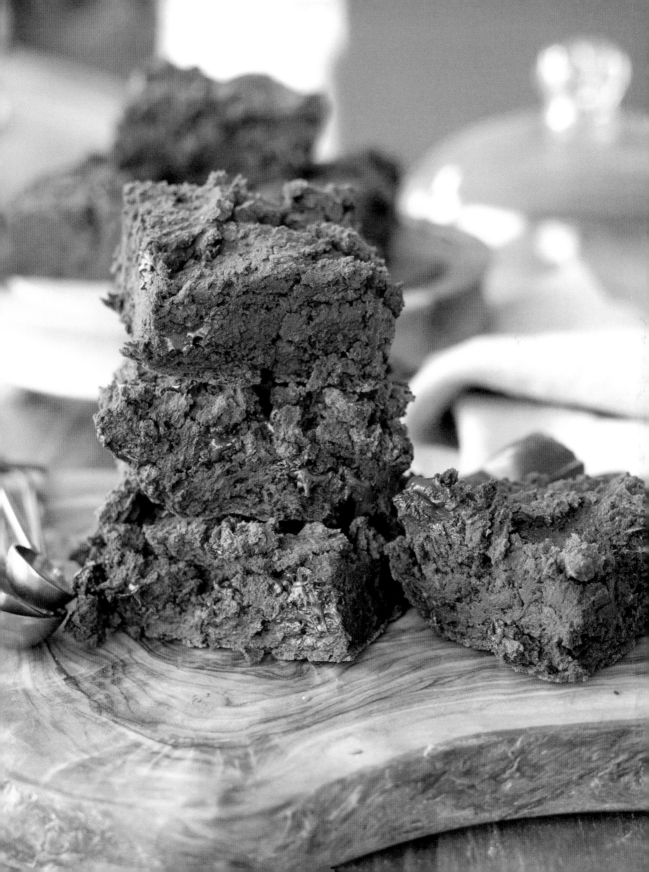

Resources

Your Body in Balance by Neal D. Barnard, MD, FACC: This is an excellent resource for understanding hormones, thyroid issues, polycystic ovary syndrome (PCOS), and more. Dr Barnard also shares research on the impact fat and other nutrients have on the body and how a low-fat, plant-based diet can help you overcome the above health concerns.

The Starch Solution by John McDougall, MD, and Mary McDougall: A great resource for understanding fat storage, protein, B_{12}, and carbohydrates on a plant-based diet, along with scientific research on these topics. It's also a great scientific resource for how to lose weight on a low-fat, high-carb diet.

The McDougall Program for Maximum Weight Loss by John A. McDougall, MD: This is another great resource for a high-carb, low-fat, plant-based diet that details the importance on how dietary fat affects weight loss, along with plate building, weight maintenance, and calorie dilution.

YouTube video by Jeff Novick, MS, RDN: "Calorie Density: How to Eat More, Weigh Less, and Live Longer." This video gives in-depth information about keeping fats low and explains the research behind sustainable weight loss using the principles of calorie density.

Acknowledgments

I'm deeply grateful to Dr. John McDougall, whose model of a plant-based diet not only transformed my life but also the lives of thousands of other people, too. His books and programs are a wonderful resource for anyone looking to improve their health, and I cannot recommend his work enough.

Index

About the Author

KIKI NELSON is known as Plantiful Kiki on social media. Born in the Yucatán, she adopted a plant-based diet after previous failed attempts to regain her health through weight loss. By combining a plant-based diet and a strategy for eating for satiation, she lost seventy pounds, and now helps others do the same.

Kiki is the co-creator of the Eat More Weigh Less Program, which has now helped thousands lose weight and keep it off. She lives in Colorado with her husband and two children and enjoys the beautiful mountains. You can learn more about Kiki on her website and connect with her and the community on all her social media platforms.

www.plantifulkiki.com

▶ Plantiful Kiki

◎ @Plantfiulkiki

♪ @Plantifulkiki

f @plantifulkiki